Kampo Treatment *for* Climacteric Disorders

A Handbook for Practitioners

Yoshiharu Shibata, M.D.
Jean Wu

Paradigm Publications ‡ Brookline, Massachusetts ‡ 1997

Kampo Treatment for Climacteric Disorders
A Handbook for Practitioners

Yoshiharu Shibata, M.D.
Jean Wu

Copyright © Paradigm Publications
44 Linden Street
Brookline, Massachusetts 02146 USA

Library of Congress Cataloging-in-Publication Data

Shibata, Yoshiharu, 1920-1993.
  Kampo treatment for climacteric disorders: a handbook for practitioners / Yoshiharu Shibata, Jean Wu
    p. cm./
  Includes bibliographical references and index.
  ISBN 0-912111-51-8
  1. Menopause--Complications--Alternative treatment. 2. Herbs--Therapeutic use--Japan. I. Wu, Jean, 1961-. II. Title.
  RG 186.S6655 1996
  618.17'75--dc21   97-4784
                                         CIP

Library of Congress Number: 97-4784
International Standard Book Number (ISBN): 0-912111-51-8
Printed in the United States of America

Distributors
AcuMedic CENTRE
101-105 CAMDEN HIGH STREET
LONDON NW1 7JN
Tel: 0171-388 5783/6704
Catalogue on Request

Table of Contents

Acknowledgements

This book would not have materialized without the help and encouragement of many. In particular, the authors would like to express their gratitude to the following people:

Mr. Yoshihiro Nagakura of the Nagakura Pharmaceutical Company, who brought the authors together and provided financial support for the research; and the staff of the Nagakura Company, especially Mr. Hai-Rin Tan, Mr. Masahiro Tanabe, Mr. Kon-ei Gan, for their suggestions and research assistance, and Mrs. Morishita for helping to find reference materials.

Dr. Keigo Nakata of the Sei Kou En Clinic, for sharing his vision of Kampo medical practice; and for his time, patience, and incisive comments.

Mr. Hiroshi Hanioka, who contributed his insights on formula application and his knowledge of classical Kampo literature.

Dan Kenner, for critiquing the first draft and helping with idea development.

Dr. Yoshiko Nakano and Dr. Yoshiro Ogata, for sharing their experience on certain clinical issues.

Dr. Michael R. Reich, Director of the Takemi Program in International Health at the Harvard School of Public Health, for his criticism and invaluable advice on the revision of the manuscript in its preliminary stages.

Dr. Charles Leslie at the Harvard Medical School Department of Social Medicine and Dr. Peter Goldman at the Harvard School of Public Health, for reading and critiquing Part I, and for their encouragement.

Dr. Harald K. Heggenhougen at the Harvard School of Public Health, for both inspiration and instruction.

Dr. Kiichiro Tsutani, who provided counsel and reference materials.

The Department of Pharmacognosy at Kyoto University; especially Dr. Aya Nitta.

Nigel Wiseman, for his technical assistance with formula names and ingredients.

Bob Felt, Martha Fielding, and the rest of the Paradigm production team.

The Gochis, Jean's host family in Kyoto.

Minoru and Maya Higashida, for providing information and samples of traditional medicines.

Frederic Tellier, who prepared and revised the tables and illustrations with unflagging good humor and was a wellspring of support.

Our families, who accommodated us throughout.

Designation

Paradigm Publications is a participant in the Council of Oriental Medical Publishers and supports their effort to inform readers of how works in Chinese medicine are prepared.

Kampo Treatment for Climacteric Disorders is an original work prepared from the studies and clinical practice of Dr. Yoshiharu Shibata. Unless noted, the English rendering of formula names follows Nigel Wiseman's ***Glossary of Chinese Medical Terms and Acupuncture Points*** and ***A Practical Dictionary of Chinese Medicine*** (see Bibliography).

User's Guide

This book presumes a basic knowledge of anatomy and physiology, and familiarity with physiological changes underlying menopause. Although much of the book has relevance to general health care, by virtue of its subject matter, it is intended for practitioners engaged in the care of older women. Since it presents the material from a Western perspective, it is primarily useful for physicians, nurses, and others trained in the biomedical tradition. But it can also be of interest to practitioners of other systems of health care who wish to explore the benefits of Oriental medicine. Acupuncturists and herbalists in the Chinese tradition may find it a useful reference, especially if they intend to collaborate with biomedical practitioners.

Part I provides background information. Chapter 1 is a general introduction. It discusses the relevance of Kampo medicine to the management of menopausal problems, and describes the scope and limitations of this manual. Chapter 2 outlines the historical development of Kampo in Japan, ending with a survey of its present status. Chapter 3 examines the major differences between Kampo and biomedicine and attempts to put into perspective some common objections to herbal remedies. Chapter 4 is an overview of the applications of Kampo within the framework of modern medicine.

Part II sets forth the rudiments of Kampo practice, from diagnosis to issues surrounding treatment and evaluation. It opens with a discussion of selected traditional concepts in Chapter 5. Diagnostics are covered in the next two chapters. Chapter 6 deals with routine diagnostic procedures. Abdominal examination, an important component of diagnosis in Kampo, is the subject of Chapter 7, which describes common abdominal signs and lays out the procedure for conducting abdominal palpation.

Chapter 8 takes up the topic of pattern identification. Since we are presuming the use of convenient commercial extract preparations rather than traditional decoctions, this presentation is geared to the limitations inherent in the modern format, discussed in Chapter 9. Chapter 10 addresses the issues of dosage, therapeutic fine-tuning, and evaluation of therapeutic response.

Chapter 11 reviews the adverse effects that have been reported on Kampo therapy and the types of situations where they arise. Chapter 12 offers a few recommendations to novice practitioners and summarizes the precautions to be taken in Kampo treatment.

Material in Part II is common to all Kampo practice. Readers should familiarize themselves with it before proceeding further.

Part III presents Kampo treatment for climacteric disorders. Each of the nine chapters in this section focuses on one aspect of common problems affecting perimenopausal women. A special feature is the quick-reference table that accompanies each chapter, designed to facilitate the identification of appropriate remedies.

Remedies introduced in this manual appear in Part IV in alphabetical order according to their English names. For each remedy, names, composition, indications, and applications are given, as well as miscellaneous notes germane to its use. Preliminary Considerations at the beginning of Part IV furnishes the information necessary for proper interpretation of the entries.

There are two appendices. Appendix A compiles a list of substances incorporated in Kampo remedies requiring prudent dispensation. Appendix B provides a list of distributors of Kampo extract preparations in the US.

To help promote a unified approach to the translation of Oriental traditional medicine, technical terms that are similar in meaning to their counterparts in Chinese medicine are standardized to Nigel Wiseman's *Glossary of Chinese Medical Terms and Points,* an authoritative work characterized by meticulous attention to linguistic detail. Names of herbs and formulas are similarly rendered according to Wiseman's *A Practical Dictionary of Chinese Medicine.*

Translation of terms with meanings peculiar to Kampo was governed primarily by their sense and intelligibility in English, not strict word-for-word correspondence. In particular, technical terms that originate from Chinese medicine but subsequently acquired a distinct significance in Kampo are rendered differently from the aforementioned Glossary. Distinction of the concepts signified thus took precedence over the preservation of possible intercontextual linguistic associations in the original Chinese as a translation criterion. For persons familiar with Chinese medicine, notes are provided where Kampo differs significantly in theory or practice from its parent system.

PART I

SKETCHES FROM THE PAST
AND PRESENT

Chapter 1
Introduction

Kampo is one of Japan's medical traditions. The term Kampo is a compound of two words: *Kan,* the old name for China; and *Hō,* meaning way or method. As may be inferred from this etymology, Kampo traces its roots to Chinese medicine, which spread through Asia, and still influences many Oriental therapeutic systems. In its broader meaning Kampo encompasses physiotherapies such as acupuncture and moxibustion. However, in present-day Japan it primarily designates pharmacotherapy derived from Chinese medicine. This is the aspect considered in this book.

Kampo is not just medicine imported from China. Like other elements of Chinese culture that filtered into Japan throughout history, it underwent transformations in the crucible of Japanese culture. To call it a distinct system would be an overstatement: the primary qualities that characterize its difference from Western medicine are more or less those identified in its Chinese progenitor. However, over the ages since its first introduction, it was continually modified to accommodate the demands, temperament, and customs peculiar to Japan and its people. In particular, reformations in the 17th and 18th centuries set its development along an evolutionary trajectory that significantly diverged from medicine in China.

The dominant modality of treatment in Japan is Western biomedicine, officially adopted as the orthodox system in the late 19th century as one of many social policies intended to promote modernization. Unlike China where the postwar development of traditional Chinese medicine was driven by government policy and an international political isolation from Western medical materials and information, Japan with its burgeoning pharmaceutical industry and large scale drug importation did not need to rely on traditional medicines for primary health care. Yet Kampo did not survive as an anachronistic cultural habit in the exclusive province of herbalists or other lay practitioners serving isolated pockets of the population. On the contrary, with the development of extract preparations of Kampo remedies in the 1950's and the approval of Kampo products for national health insurance coverage in the 1970's, it became an increasing aspect of modern Japanese medical practice. Popular demand has been an important driving force behind this resurgence.

Presently, Japanese physicians are exploring the use of Kampo to deal with the consequences of an epidemiological shift from acute infectious diseases to chronic degenerative conditions, as well as the comorbidity that attends an aging population. Kampo medicine causes few adverse effects and is suitable for long-term administration. A single remedy can often address multiple diseases. In addition, Kampo's emphasis on a patient's subjective complaints makes it particularly relevant in today's health care, where quality of life has become an important issue.

The experience of the Japanese, as they grapple with the meaningful integration of traditional medicine, could be eminently instructive for the West. A dialogue of exchange has already begun between investigators in Japan and Europe. Yet Kampo remains virtually unknown in the US, save among a limited circle of acupuncturists who have access to training or information from Japan. This book was born out of the desire to introduce the contemporary applications of Kampo to our colleagues in the biomedical community, in hope of initiating a cross-fertilization that will promote humanistic and holistic medical practices.

Constrained by limited time and resources, we elected to focus our undertaking on the subject of climacteric or menopausal syndrome, a multi-faceted entity that bears upon many women's health issues as well as some common chronic conditions that affect the general population. As such, it affords a cross-sectional illustration of the Kampo approach. In effect, this text is a "slice" of Japanese medical practice in which Kampo plays a significant role.

It is also a timely topic. During the past thirty years we have witnessed a significant change in the status of menopause in the West. From a minor issue of nuisance complaints, it has become a vital concern in the care of older women.(1) Part of the reason for this revision is the development of a new medical model of the climacteric. This model interprets the transition from the childbearing to the nonchildbearing phase of a woman's life as an endocrinopathy, an estrogen deficiency disease with far-reaching deleterious effects.(2,3) Another reason for this conceptual evolution is demographic. The mean age of menopause is 50 years. About one-third (39 million) of women in the U.S. are 45 years old or older. They have an average life expectancy of 81 years. Perimenopausal women are thus an ever growing part of the population.(4,5) The sheer size of these numbers compels examination of issues around menopause and a search for safer, more effective treatment of the problems related to it.

Although medical opinion has undergone wide vacillations, estrogen replacement therapy is currently considered the treatment of choice for menopausal disorders. It is indicated for relief of neuroendocrine changes and for the prevention of urogenital atrophy, osteoporosis, and atherosclerotic cardiovascular disease. With an increasing focus on the latter long-term goals, many physicians are now advocating the routine use of estrogen.(6)

Yet hormone therapy is not the only solution. Nor is it the best choice in many cases. Nonhormonal measures can have a positive impact on the health and wellbeing of climacteric and postmenopausal women. Kampo is one such alternative. Its concern with individual variations is especially pertinent to climacteric disorders, where there is great variation of symptoms among patients. Many gynecologists in Japan consider it to be a good substitute or addition to a conventional treatment regimen. According to a recent survey, among 70% of Japanese gynecologists who utilize Kampo, 90% prescribe it for their climacteric patients.(7)

Regardless of Japanese practice, a critical look at Kampo and other nonhormonal measures is important for the following reasons:

1. Adverse effects of hormone replacement therapy.

2. Poor compliance with hormone replacement therapy.

3. Women's preferences.

1. Hormone replacement therapy (HRT): Side effects, risks, and contraindications

The common side effects of estrogen therapy include breast tenderness, irregular bleeding, edema and bloating, nausea, vomiting, and headaches. Progestogen, which is added to estrogen to prevent endometrial hyperplasia in women with an intact uterus, causes withdrawal bleeding and can induce premenstrual-like dysphoria, lower abdominal cramps, and dysmenorrhea. Some types of progestogen are androgenic, giving rise to acne, hirsutism, and deepening of voice.(8) It has also been suggested that certain progestogens can negate the beneficial impact of estrogen on lipid profiles.(9)

The risks of HRT outweigh its benefits for women with certain pre-existing conditions. Absolute contraindications include estrogen-dependent neoplasia, active or recurrent thromboembolic disease, acute liver disease; and recent myocardial infarction, cerebrovascular accident, or transient ischemic attack. Relative contraindications include a strong family history of breast cancer, chronic liver or gallbladder disease, diabetes mellitus, hypertension, hyperlipidemia, endometriosis, fibroids, and migraine headaches.(4) According to a survey of primary care providers, many physicians do not readily prescribe HRT for fear of inducing or aggravating cancer, hypertension, and thrombosis.(10)

2. Poor compliance

Poor patient compliance poses a serious problem in hormone therapy. Studies have shown that many women receiving oral HRT took the medication only sporadically. Some discontinued because of side effects. Others never had their prescriptions filled because they were not fully convinced of the benefits and safety of HRT.(8,11) Thus actual, anticipated, or feared side effects render HRT unacceptable to a significant number of women.

3. Women's preference for natural treatment options

The generation of women entering the climacteric phase of their lives today want to be actively involved in the decisions regarding their health. Reflecting the influence of the holistic health movement, many prefer alternative modes of therapy over HRT for alleviation of menopausal complaints. In a 1985 study undertaken to assess attitudes toward menopause, 64% of the 233 respondents endorsed agreement with the statement, "Natural approaches are better than estrogen replacement therapy." 30% were undecided, and only 6% disagreed.(12)

Kampo remedies may well answer women's demand for a safe natural medicine. They consist of natural substances whose therapeutic benefits have been explored and documented through 2000 years of human experiment in the Orient. The substances are blended into formulas, each with a distinct spectrum of actions. One formula can often ameliorate climacteric problems as well as pre-existing conditions. More than 40 are in common use for this purpose. Knowledgeable doctors may "fine-tune" a standard formula by adding or deleting component substances, or devise new combinations to tailor treatment to individual needs.

Lack of scientific evidence is the common barrier to acceptance faced by every therapeutic tradition outside of the modern orthodoxy. Kampo is no exception. Though theoretically possible, the application of modern standards of clinical investigation to the evaluation of Kampo therapies raises many unresolved methodological issues. Past policies and regulations in Japan have provided little incentive for the Kampo pharmaceutical industry to sponsor quality clinical studies. However, the situation has changed recently. New Kampo medications are now subjected to essentially the same regulations as are Western drugs. More importantly, re-evaluation of formulas that were approved in the past has been initiated by the Japanese Ministry of Health and Welfare. Both the quality and quantity of studies are expected to increase as a result but, thus far, good clinical studies are the exception rather than the rule.(13)

The lack of conclusive statistical proof is mitigated by basic research of numerous traditional medicinal materials employed in Kampo, which has demonstrated beyond a doubt that there is a sound scientific basis for their use. The test of time and the corpus of clinical case studies that have been accruing in modern Japan also weigh in Kampo's favor. As informal testimonies to Kampo's safety and efficacy, the latter may be dismissed as folkloric or anecdotal. However, together with basic research, historical and modern experience constitute a body of positive and provocative data that deserves more in-depth investigation.

It is not the purpose of this book to prove that Kampo works. Rather, within the modest scope of a handbook for practitioners, we have confined ourselves largely to a elementary presentation of the Classical style of Kampo *(Kohōha)* which has characterized mainstream practice in modern times. Its preparation drew directly from the more than four decades of Kampo practice of a physician author. In the spirit of consensus-seeking, we also consulted a selection of textbooks, manuals, and articles written by other Kampo physicians and medical and pharmaceutical researchers.

This work is thus more than a record of one physician's understanding and clinical experience. Although the content is necessarily shaped by the authors' judgement, what emerged from our efforts to exclude idiosyncrasies reflects a general consensus concerning current Classical-style practice; in particular, what physicians considered to be the responsible use of commercial extract preparations.

Our decision to portray the Classical practice in no way negates the importance or achievements of other currents of Kampo. We believe that several features of Classical Kampo render it more readily useful in the Western framework. One of these features is its practical clinical orientation. This means minimal theory, with a relatively small number of broad concepts guiding clinical thought. Though we have pared these theories further to a level appropriate for this work, there nonetheless remain several concepts that are useful for expanding the biomedical model. Thus this work should appeal to practitioners who find the existing literature of Oriental medicine too opaque in its theoretical orientation. In terms of diagnostic technique, the abdominal palpation favored in the Classical tradition is easier to learn than the pulse diagnosis emphasized in Chinese medicine and other schools of Kampo. Classical practice also centers on the application of a limited number of remedies, which are a manageable addition to the modern physician's therapeutic repertory.

In describing traditional medical concepts, we did not go back to the primary classical sources but took the generally accepted contemporary interpretations as given. Indications for the remedies were likewise based on a contemporary exegeses of traditional indications.

Formulas are the basic unit of Kampo therapy. The approximately 60 formulas appearing in this book mostly derive from the Classical tradition. Virtually all are common Kampo remedies for which extract preparations are readily available. The book does not explicate the properties of individual herbs, and deals with the adjustment of formulas to a very limited extent. To begin to understand why the formulas act as they do and how to modify them, readers must turn to a study of traditional materia medica and recent pharmacological research.

There is a dearth of information on Kampo practice in English. Unlike the few volumes that do exist, this book is specifically designed to make the subject more accessible to Western clinicians, and to facilitate the application of Kampo within the existing biomedical framework. In the choice of terminology, we adopted modern parlance whenever this made sense. In the description and interpretation of traditional medical concepts, we made frequent references to modern medicine. In general, we have noted links and differences between the two systems while implying no absolute equivalance.

Above all, we have taken great pains in the structure and organization of the material. Partly because unifying principles differ across time and culture and partly because Classical practice de-emphasizes systematic theory, the source material can at times resemble rambling lists. We have tried to capture such lists in categories where possible. Since intelligibility to Western readers is a primary concern, we often found it necessary to depart from the manner by which Kampo is typically presented by Japanese for a Japanese audience. This is particularly true in our presentation of abdominal examination and the indications for Kampo remedies.

We also wish to acknowledge the inherent inadequacy of the book format. Traditionally, medicine is an art that is passed on from a master to disciples. Even today in Japan, apprenticeship with an established Kampo physician is the way to mastery. Yet for students of Oriental healing arts in the West, books often must serve as the principal conduit of knowledge. The intricacies of therapy cannot really be boiled down to tidy rules suitable for written presentation. Especially in a simplified introductory manual such as this, many finer points are not addressed. Nevertheless, we believe that the guidelines here provided will help to induct a beginner into Kampo practice.

Finally, it is our hope that by delineating ways Japanese physicians are blending tradition with modern science in the service of patients, this book will pique the curiosity of thoughtful investigators in the West and help to stimulate research and clinical trials on Kampo therapy in the U.S., not only for menopause, but also in other areas of application.

References for Chapter 1

(1) Judd, Howard and Wulf H. Utian. "Introduction: What We Hope to Learn" (presented at the symposium, Current Perspectives in the Management of the Menopausal and Postmenopausal Patient, 1986). *American Journal of Obstetrics and Gynecology* 156 (1987): 1279-80.

(2) Hunter, Myra S. "Emotional Well-Being, Sexual Behaviour and Hormone Replacement Therapy." *Maturitas* 12 (1990): 299-314

(3) Utian, Wulf H. "Overview on Menopause." *American Journal of Obstetrics and Gynecology* 156 (1987): 1280-3.

(4) Notelovitz, Morris. "Estrogen Replacement Therapy: Indications, Contraindications and Agent Selection." *American Journal of Obstetrics and Gynecology* 161 (1989): 1832-41.

(5) Utian, Wulf H. "Biosynthesis and Physiologic Effects of Estrogen and Pathophysiologic Effects of Estrogen Deficiency: A Review." *American Journal of Obstetrics and Gynecology* 161 (1989): 1828-31.

(6) Koster, A. "Hormone Replacement Therapy: Use Patterns in 51-Year-Old Danish Women." *Maturitas* 12 (1990): 345-356.

(7) Tanabe, Isao. "Kampōyaku wa Kiku Ka (Does Kampo Medicine Work?)." *Asahi Shinbunsha*, 1988, p.78.

(8) Hahn, Ricardo G. "Complicance Considerations with Estrogen Replacement: Withdrawal Bleeding and Other Factors." *American Journal of Obstetrics and Gynecology* 161 (1989): 1854-8

(9) Hirvonen, E., M. Malkonen, V. Manninen. "Effect of Different Progestogens on Lipoproteins during Postmenopausal Replacement Therapy." *New England Journal of Medicine* 304 (1981): 560-563.

(10) Holzman, G.B., Ravitch, M.M., Metheny, W. *et al.* "Physicians' Judgements about Estrogen Replacement Therapy for Menopausal Women." *Obstetrics and Gynecology* 63 (1984): 303-11.

(11) Ravnikar, V.A. "Compliance with Hormone Therapy." *American Journal of Obstetrics and Gynecology* 156 (1984): 1332-4.

(12) Leiblum, Sandra R. and Leora C. Swartzman. "Women's Attitudes about the Menopause: An Update." *Maturitas* 81 (1986): 47-56.

(13) Tsutani, Kiichiro. "On the Evaluation of Herbal Medicines, an East Asian Perspective: Current Status of Clinical Studies of Herbal Medicines in China and Japan." Research Paper No.60, Oct. 1991, Takemi program in International Health, Harvard School of Public Health.

Chapter 2
History

The evolution of Kampo from Chinese medicine and its diffusion in Japan are rich topics that bear examination in their own right. They have been described in greater detail by other authors.[1] The following brief historical overview is intended to lend some perspective to the Kampo practice introduced in this book.

I. Early period

Chinese medicine first came to Japan by way of Korea in the 5th century. Direct exchanges began in the 7th century. Emissaries were dispatched to study medicine in China, and medical books and crude drugs began to arrive in Japan in a steady flow. In the beginning of the 8th century, medical education and practice modeled on the Tang Dynasty system were established to serve the aristocracy.

Attempts were made to render the imported Chinese works more accessible to the Japanese. The year 984 marked the completion of *Ishinpo*, compiled from more than 100 Chinese sources from the Sui (581-618) and Tang (618-907) dynasties. Far from being a translation of randomly selected materials, it reflects the effort of the author to extract and organize information according to his own insight. For several hundred years it remained the most influential work.

II. 10th to 15th century

The main trend continued to be the introduction and diffusion of Chinese medicine, in which Buddhist monks played a major part. However, important developments in Chinese medicine between the 12th and 14th century remained virtually unknown, and Chinese medical theories in general failed to root in Japan.

---

[1] *See, for example, "Chinese Traditional Medicine in Japan" by Y. Otsuka, in Leslie, Charles, ed. Asian Medical Systems, Berkeley: University of California Press, 1976, pp.322-340; and Lock, Margaret. East Asian Medicine in Urban Japan, Berkeley: University of California Press, 1980.*

III. 16th to mid-19th century

In the 16th century, due to the endeavors of Manase Dōsan (1507-1594), Kampo acquired a theoretical framework adapted from Chinese medicine of the Jin and Yuan periods, and developed into a comprehensive system of diagnosis and treatment based on disease pattern identification.

Dōsan's system spread throughout Japan[2] and was continually revised and simplified to suit the needs of local practitioners and to incorporate the influx of Ming period texts from China. In spite of the modifications, this system of medicine still contained elements that appeared too speculative for many leading physicians of the day. Deriving impetus from a restoration movement in Confucianism, a reform movement was launched in the medical circles in the second half of the 17th century. Reformers criticized the prevailing system for having lapsed into metaphysics and called for the restoration of a medicine grounded in clinical observation. The system was to be organized anew based upon Chinese medicine as revealed in original, more ancient texts.

The principal work extolled by the reformers was Zhang Zhong Jing's *Treatise on Cold Damage (Shang Han Lun),* a text from the later Han period (c.220 A.D.) which sets forth the treatment for cold-induced or febrile disorders; and *Essential Prescriptions of the Golden Coffer (Jin Gui Yao Lue),* its companion volume on miscellanous diseases. Discovered by the Japanese medical circle in 1659, this work became the object of intense research and study. On account of their emphasis on the classics, proponents of this movement were named the Classical School *(Kohōha),* and the medical order they spurned as corrupt came to be known as the Neoteric School *(Goseiha).*

The reform movement did not stop at the return to the classics. As the most radical embodiment of the movement's positivist leaning, Yoshimasu Tōdō (1702-1773) went so far as to advocate thoretical nihilism. For Tōdō, the answer was the creation of a therapeutic system anchored in empiricism, divested of all prevailing theories of physiology, pathology, and herbal medicine.

Principally from the aforementioned work of Zhang Zhong Jing, Tōdō distilled a system of lock-and-key correspondences between patterns of symptoms and signs and remedies to treat them. In Chinese medicine and the Neoteric tradition, diagnosis and determination of treatment are divided into distinct stages: Starting with a constellation of clinical findings, the practitioner identifies a pattern of pathologies, decides upon the proper method of treatment, and subsequently devises a suitable remedy. Tōdō's therapeutics forged a direct link between the observed pattern of symptoms and signs and the choice of remedy, eliminating the intermediate steps which relied on theories. It is in effect a return to the earlier days when Chinese medicine lacked a comprehensive theoretical structure. Tōdō also emphasized abdominal palpation over pulse palpation, an important departure from the parent Chinese system and a bias persisting to this day.[3]

---

[2] *But mainly in the urban centers and among the elites, limited availability of the Chinese materia medica being one major barrier to its popularization until recent times.*

[3] *Tōdō's other extremist ideas and practices are evoked today only as medical curiosities and are not mentioned here.*

After Tōdō, many variations on his views appeared within the Classical School. Efforts were made to reinstate a limited number of traditional concepts in the theoretical vacuum left by the radical reformist. Contemporary Kampo is very much a progeny of this fortified version of Tōdō's therapeutic system, with remedies from Zhang Zhong Jing's work (little used nowadays in China) still forming the core of its therapeutics. It might be said that, because of the endeavors of the Classical School, Kampo first became distinctly and truly Japanese.

The Neoteric School, though eclipsed by the Classical School, did not phase out of existence. Its practices are carried on by unbroken generations of disciples. Today, it is still a significant current in Kampo.

From the late 18th century on, various eclectic sects (dubbed Setchūha, the Syncretic School) appeared on the scene. Each made free use of the perceived strengths of the two foregoing schools. As European medicine gradually became ascendant in Japan, a number of physicians also attempted to weld a global medicine out of Kampo and Western medicine.[4]

IV. Second half of 19th century to 1950

Kampo entered a period of rapid decline as the tide of modernization advanced under the Meiji government (1868-1912). Having decided to adopt the German medical system in 1874, the government enacted a series of measures that successively excluded traditional medicine from medical training and qualifying examinations, culminating in a law passed in 1883 which deprived existing Kampo practitioners of their legal standing as medical doctors.

In ever dwindling numbers, Kampo doctors continued to practice privately in response to popular demand. By the end of the 19th century, however, they had virtually disappeared from the medical scene. The tradition was kept alive at the grass-roots level primarily by pharmacists and sellers of traditional medicines.

A notable consequence of modernization was that traditional medicines as a potential source of modern drugs became one of the main topics of research at Japanese universities. Research into the chemistry and pharmacology of substances used in Kampo began to demonstrate the scientific basis underlying their use. The best known fruit of these early endeavors was the isolation of ephedrine from *Ephedra sinica.* Thus even as Kampo receded into twilight, a scientific foundation contributing to its revival was being laid.

In time, proponents of Kampo began to rise from the ranks of physicians trained under the Western system. 1934 marked the founding of the Japan Society for Kampo Medicine. Composed of physicians and pharmacists interested in Kampo research and practice, the society had as one of its primary goals the modernization of Kampo. A training program was established. Teaching materials in modern Japanese incorporating modern medical terminology were developed.

---

[4] *This is also when the traditional medical system came to be called Kampō (the way or method of the Han), to distinguish it from Rampō (the way or method of the Ran, or Dutch).*

These laid the foundation for modern Kampo education. In 1941, the torch bearers of the extant schools collaborated in writing a text on Kampo therapy. Later revised extensively, it played an instrumental role in the spread of Kampo.[5]

World War II brought these first attempts at revival to a halt.

V. Modern period (1950 to date)

The revival movement resumed after the war. A number of organizations were formed to promote Kampo and other aspects of traditional Oriental medicine. Kampo medicine also entered a new era. Methods for large-scale production of herbal extracts at reduced pressure and temperature were developed. In the 1950s, several pharmaceutical companies began to manufacture and market modern extract preparations of traditional formulas. Availability of easy-to-administer extracts not only brought convenience for consumers but also facilitated research on Kampo medicine.

Yet it was not until the 1970s when Kampo succeeded in gaining a measure of recognition in the general medical community. Sensational publicity about acupuncture anesthesia performed in China created a surge in public interest in traditional medicine. In 1976, petitioning by patient groups and the political support of key physicians prompted the Ministry of Health and Welfare to approve a number of extract preparations of Kampo formulas for coverage by the national health insurance. The list of approved extracts has since grown to include about 150 formulas.[6]

This development proved to be a mixed blessing. On the one hand, it promoted the use of Kampo and turned out to be of pivotal importance to Kampo's entry into modern medical practice. Of all physicians who utilize some form of Kampo, the majority began after extracts were covered by national health insurance. On the other hand, inclusion in the national health insurance system slowed the impetus to carry out quality research on Kampo.

Since physicians in Japan can dispense drugs, one might suppose that economic incentive plays a part in physicians' use of Kampo. A 1986 survey conducted by the Japan Society for Oriental Medicine asked its physician members what motivated them to take up Kampo therapy. By far the most frequently cited reason was the quest for safe and effective new therapeutic methods (43% of the 1877 answers given by 1246 respondents). Some were motivated after attending lectures or seminars on Kampo (17%). Not infrequently, Kampo entered into physicians' practice after they themselves or members of their families tried the traditional remedies with favorable outcomes (18%). By contrast, wishes of the patient was low on the list (3%), following disappointment with modern medicine (8%) and learning about Kampo through colleagues or at meetings of medical society (4%).

---

[5] Ātsuka, Keisetsu, Y. Dōmei, S. Totaro et al. *Kampo Dai Iten (A Comprehensive Textbook of Kampo Medicine)*. Tokyo: Kōdansha, 1975.

[6] *That the majority of formulas approved for coverage come from the Treatise on Cold Damage and the Essential Prescriptions of the Golden Coffer reflects the relative dominance of the Classical school influence since the 1930's revival of Kampo medicine.*

Approximately half of all Japanese physicians practice some form of Kampo. The majority use Kampo extracts adjunctively to Western biomedicine. The disease profile of the patients they treat is similar to that of patients treated by physicians who practice biomedicine exclusively. A small minority (estimated to be less than 4%) specialize in Kampo. Patients they care for mainly suffer from allergic, autoimmune, or functional disorders.

Within the medical community, the use of Kampo is most conspicuous in obstetrics and gynecology. According to a 1985 study, about 70% of the 2479 gynecologists surveyed reported using Kampo medicines. The 10 top conditions cited were (in order of frequency):

1. climacteric syndrome/ovarian deficiency syndrome
2. nonspecific complaints
3. infertility
4. dysmenorrhea
5. ovulatory disorders
6. problems during pregnancy (such as influenza, constipation, vomiting, toxemia)
7. postoperative recovery
8. benign tumors
9. malignant tumors
10. infections

Perhaps nothing else gives a better indication of the spread of Kampo than the phenomenal growth of the Kampo pharmaceutical market itself. From 1976-89, sales of Kampo medicines grew more than 15-fold, while sales of other drugs increased only 2.6 fold. Kampo products now account for nearly 3% of total Japanese drug expenditure (about 166 billion yen in 1990).[7] The sale of over-the-counter Kampo medicines is no longer confined to traditional herbal pharmacies. It is estimated that approximately 3/4 of 74,000 pharmacies nationwide carry one or more brands of Kampo extract preparations.[8]

Research and education

Many societies are active in the promotion of Kampo medicine. They sponsor symposiums, conduct research, and publish periodicals and newsletters. The principal one is the Japan Society for Oriental Medicine, whose research activities encompass all fields of Oriental medicine. Its membership has multiplied from 94 in 1950 to 10,300 in 1991. Since the 1970's, a number of public and private Oriental medicine research centers have been established in Japan, some of which are part of noted schools of medicine or pharmacy. Research is also carried out at universities and privately by the pharmaceutical companies.

Since the medical reform law passed by the Meiji government remains in effect, only licensed biomedical doctors can legally practice Kampo.[9] Any who aspire to a career in Kampo medicine must go through a curriculum of studies

---

[7] *Statistics from the Official Bulletin of Pharmaceutical Affairs, published by the Pharmaceutical Affairs Bureau of the Japanese Ministry of Health and Welfare, 1992.*
[8] *Survey conducted in 1991 by the Yakkyoku Shinbun Sha.*
[9] *Pharmacists are allowed to prescribe and dispense Kampo medications, but not to perform diagnostic palpation.*

and training equivalent to Western medical education. As yet, no educational institution offers training and professional degrees in Kampo medicine, though it is gradually gaining a foothold in the curriculum of medical, dental, and pharmaceutical colleges throughout Japan. The trend is most pronounced among pharmaceutical colleges. Among the 80 medical colleges, a mere handful have introduced instruction in traditional medicine; and only one, the Toyama Medical and Pharmaceutical University, offers a course that includes clinical training. Consequently, interested students must depend on methods other than formal medical education. Many form study groups or clubs, or are self-taught.

The mainstay of Kampo education is conducted at a postgraduate level, in the form of hundreds of seminars held by various societies and local medical and pharmaceutical associations each year. Many of these seminars are sponsored by Kampo extract manufacturers, who also organize lectures and training courses of their own for physicians and pharmacists. In addition, programs for physicians are offered by a number of institutes promoting the research and use of Oriental medicine.

Books and journals are an important means of diffusion. More than 30 periodicals on Kampo medicine exist. Some 360 books were published between 1978-1983, a 1.7-fold increase over the previous 10-year span. The number of publications continues to rise. They range from books for the lay readership to erudite treatises directed at specialists.

Because of the lack of a standard course of training, there is wide disparity in the sophistication of Kampo practice among physicians. Some rely only on elementary-level handbooks or pamphlets distributed by Kampo extract makers. Many use extract preparations in the manner of biomedical drugs to counter specific disease entities, with little regard for traditional injunctions. Iatrogenic problems have arisen due to such unfortunate "rationalization" of traditional medicine.

That Kampo practitioners are themselves physicians is often held up as a desirable feature of traditional medical practice in Japan. Presumably, doctors can evaluate Kampo from the standpoint of biomedical science and make discriminating use of the two systems. However, this potential advantage cannot be realized to a significant extent until Kampo is integrated into regular medical education. Indeed, as long as Kampo remains subordinate, its very cooptation by the biomedical establishment may threaten its preservation.

Styles of Practice

Contemporary Kampo does not present a unified front, but is rather a spectrum formed by the interplay of several styles of practice. In addition to the Classical, Neoteric and Syncretic schools, a new movement based on the version of traditional Chinese medicine (TCM) presently sanctioned by the Chinese government has emerged and has been gathering momentum since the 1970's. TCM-motived development is perhaps the most active current in Kampo today. Distinctions between schools are only relative. In a sense, all Japanese physicians who utilize Kampo are Syncretists having various approaches to the combination of Kampo and biomedicine. Nevertheless, in the absence of clear biomedical criteria for the application of Kampo remedies, orientation to a traditional style remains the most prudent course.

The legacy of the Classical School still distinguishes Japanese Kampo from branches of Chinese medicine elsewhere. To its critics, this legacy is marred by its lack of a coherent theoretical structure and heavy reliance on established remedies, thus representing an impediment to the advancement of Kampo medicine. Yet, in the interest of easing access to Oriental medicine, these defects can be considered to have a meritorious aspect. For as its apologists are quick to point out, the unique contribution of the Classical School consists in the flexible, maximal use of a small corpus of remedies to cover most ordinary therapeutic needs. Classical-style application of these remedies requires minimal knowledge of traditional theories and stresses a diagnostic technique that is relatively easy to learn. In sum, this style of Kampo can constitute a feasible as well as invaluable addition to the modern physician's practice; and despite its inadequacies, provide a heuristic point of entry into Oriental pharmacotherapy.

References for Chapter 2

(1) Yakazu, Dōmei. "The Role of Education in the Revival of Traditional Medicine in Japan," Annex 6.4 in *Report: Regional Workshop on Training in Traditional Medicine,* WHO Regional Office for the Western Pacific, 1987

(2) Yasui, Hiromichi. "Nihon ni okeru Tōyō Igaku no Genkyō" (The Present Status of Oriental Medicine in Japan). In Hiroshi Sakaguchi *et al.* ed. *Proceedings of the 4th International Congress of Oriental Medicine.* Publishing Bureau of the 4th International Congress of Oriental Medicine, 1986, pp.5-16.

(3) Yasui, Hiromichi. "Kampō Igaku no Rekishi" (The History of Kampo Medicine). In Toyohiko Kikutani *et al.,* ed. *Kampō Hoken Shinryō Shishen.* Japan Society of Oriental Medicine, 1986. pp.7-12.

(4) Tanabe, Isao. "Kampōyaku wa Kiku Ka (Does Kampo Medicine Work?)". *Asahi Shinbunsha,* 1988, pp.12-17, 78-82, 226-227.

Chapter 3
Divergence from Biomedicine

Kampo is a medical system rooted in a holistic perception of existence. A sign or symptom is interpreted in the context of the individual, whose health and disease is likewise not considered in isolation, but in relation to the environment.

I. Health and disease

The idea of harmony, or balance between opposing tendencies, is central to the Kampo concept of health. The state of health is determined by balance among physiologic processes, between mind and body, and between the individual and the environment. It is a dynamic equilibrium, consisting of continual interaction and adjustment among internal and external factors.

Disease, on the other hand, is a state of disharmony or imbalance. It occurs when the innate mechanisms that restore balance are overwhelmed or disrupted. Easy susceptibility to illness is itself an imbalance. Notable among this type of imbalance are states of chronic subhealth encompassing lack of energy, lowered resistance, diminished physical and mental efficiency, and decreased capacity to adapt. Since a person in such states can easily contract more serious disorders, they are given much attention in Kampo.

II. Diagnosis and treatment

In modern medicine, diagnosis aims to identify the disease entity. Myriad analytic tests and devices aid the physician's attempt to penetrate the veil of clinical findings and disclose underlying pathologies and causative agents. The reality of disease is seen to reside in lesions and detectable physiologic disturbances, and the significance of subjective complaints tends to be discounted unless they have a truth value furnished by laboratory findings. In principle, once a diagnosis is established, a treatment regimen is devised upon additional considerations of the stage of disease, concurrent conditions, age and other individual factors, and therapeutic options. Diagnosis and treatment thus are related in a tandem fashion.

In Kampo, the thrust of diagnosis is to discern a particular pattern in the idiosyncratic expression of the illness. In a process that begins and ends with human interaction, a Kampo practitioner coalesces signs and symptoms as well as the patient's traits and propensities, and evaluates each in the light of the totality. Patient complaints are given primary attention. Moreover, in Kampo each pattern is correlated with a remedy, so that a pattern diagnosed directly indicates a specific treatment. In other words, Kampo diagnosis and treatment accomplishes in one step what in biomedicine is divided into two distinct procedures.

III. Therapeutic aims

The goal of Kampo treatment is to restore balance as well as to relieve distressing symptoms through pharmacotherapy. Predicated upon the existence of innate healing mechanisms, therapy seeks above all to support these, or remove impediments to their manifestation. The fundamental orientation is thus the restoration of health, not simply the elimination of specific disease-causing agents.

The therapeutic principle of supplementation, or building up of general vitality and host defense, deserves special mention. This principle is visible in the Western tradition of herbal medicine (witness the diverse tonics and alteratives). Yet it is conspicuously lacking in modern pharmacotherapy, apart from the recognition that disorders stemming from a lack of known essential body chemicals such as vitamins may be treated by supplying the missing entities, and that vaccines can be given to protect the body against specific infectious diseases.

Like the illness it is designed to treat, treatment is not static, but must change when the pattern of imbalance changes. Thus it involves continual reassessment of the patient and adjustment of the therapy.

IV. Preventive medicine

Kampo pattern diagnosis is based on the senses, relying on intuitive and subjective information. This bias in turn means that disorders can often be recognized at an early stage, where vague subjective complaints cannot yet be correlated with objective measurements. The attention given to susceptibility to disease and treatment to build up general vitality and immunity also bespeak the recognition that good health is the best protection against disease. As such, Kampo comes closer to true preventive medicine than modern biomedicine.

V. Characteristics of Kampo pharmacology

The traditional materia medica are all unrefined natural products, most often of plant origin, but also of mineral or animal derivation. They are typically dried or further processed to enhance the therapeutic benefits.

A. Refined drug vs. whole plant extracts

Whole plant extracts are chemically complex and difficult (if not impossible with the present methodology) to characterize pharmacologically. Sources of supply are limited. Furthermore, the chemical composition of the plant varies depending on the growing conditions, time of harvest, and storage conditions. The potency is thus non-uniform.

The aim in the West has been to isolate the ostensibly active principles, ascertain their pharmacology, and attempt to synthesize them or more potent derivatives, which are then used in place of the natural material. In other words, the natural materials are considered no more than a potential source of molecular structures for drugs.

Yet it would be a mistake to assume that the purified principles encapsulate the range of actions of the original substance. Ephedra is not just ephedrine, a nonspecific bronchodilator and nasal decongestant. The herb is employed in bronchial asthma, febrile conditions, and rheumatic disorders, but only in patients with particular characteristics. As well, ginsenoside saponins have demonstrable pharmacological properties that cannot wholly account for the clinical effects of ginseng.

The ostensibly inactive components may have valuable actions of their own, or act to amplify or temper the effects of the primary active ingredients. They may escape notice for a variety of reasons. Some are present in too small quantities or are unstable in the isolation procedures. Some may become active only after being metabolized, when the state of body chemical equilibrium favor their conversion. Other compounds may have little demonstrable effect of their own when administered alone. Constituents may also be labeled as inactive because the effects they produce are not immediate, but observable only after continuous long-term administration.

Seemingly useless or undesirable components can actually function as built-in safeguards. To wit, inert material bound with the active chemicals inhibit quick release of the latter into the blood stream. Mildly toxic compounds can signal overdose before the toxic dose of a therapeutic but highly poisonous principle is reached. Digitalis leaf is a case in point. When the leaf is given in large enough amounts for heart failure, certain components in the leaf associated with the cardiotonic principles irritate the stomach and cause nausea and vomiting. This alerts the practitioner to reduce the dosage and avoid the occurrence of more serious adverse effects. If the drug digitalis consisting of only the cardiotonic principles is used, then the first sign of overdose is directly atrial arrhythmia.(1)

Pure chemicals are justly valued for their potency. On the other hand, their use entails greater risks. Unintended actions are delivered as purely as desired actions, and the safety margin between therapeutic and toxic dosage is narrowed. The intrinsic risks are amplified by errors and inappropriate practices that can and do arise in prescription writing and administration. Not surprisingly, refined drugs are the leading cause of iatrogenic illness.(2)

Purity can also have unintended long-term consequences with respect to the pathogens. Antibiotics have created resistant bacteria, not simply because they select for strains immune to their effects, but also because it is easier for microorganisms to adapt to a single unvaried drug mechanism than to complex natural antibiotics which may work via multiple mechanisms.

The use of refined rugs overrides the difficulty of natural variation and unknown constituents associated with whole plant extracts. However, doctors who prescribe the drugs often know little about them.(2) There is something inconsistent in condemning herbal preparations on the grounds of incomplete knowledge when, in practice, doctors are ill-informed of the characteristics and interactions of the drugs they use, which is tantamount to using substances with unknown effects. This is not to suggest that current practice justifies the use of herbal medicine without further investigation. But most herbal preparations with their intrinsically larger safety margin are more tolerant of ill-informed use and the fallibility of human judgement, especially when backed by a historical record of human safety.

B. Formulas

In Kampo, a natural substance is rarely employed by itself; usually between four to ten are combined in formulas. Archeological evidence suggests that the earliest formulas were very simple and increased in complexity with the accumulation of clinical knowledge and the refinement of medical theories.

A formula containing many herbs is not to be confused with polypharmacy. Polypharmacy has been defined to be "the prescribing of multiple medications [which] creates a risk that is greater than the sum of risks from the individual drugs, because the chemistry of their interactions creates new dangers."(3) In polypharmacy, the drug-to-drug interactions are unknown or unintended. This can give rise to duplicate effects, contradictory interventions, or outright toxicity. The effect on the patient from drug incompatibility may be serious, even fatal.

In contrast, a Kampo formula is intended to function as a therapeutic unit. It has a therapeutic "personality" of its own, created expressly for a particular pattern of imbalance. Mainstream practice in Japan relies primarily on classical formulas, which might be regarded as widely tried and evaluated multi-component pharmaceuticals.[1] Each established formula has a unique name and consists of a particular group of substances in specified proportions.[2]

The rationales for combining herbs are largely similar to arguments for combining drugs. First, the effects of a single herb may be too drastic or too weak for the desired purpose. Second, combining herbs that affect different symptom profiles affords a broader spectrum of treatment, and permits clinicians to simultaneously deal with associated symptoms that frequently occur together. Further,

---

[1] *In Chinese medicine, formulas tend to be made up as needed. This approach allows one to treat imbalances not dealt with in the classics, and is theoretically superior to using established combinations. To do this properly, the practitioner is guided by clinical experience as well as a body of empirical knowledge crystallized in theories of herbal properties and elaborate rules governing herbal combination. For novices and less seasoned practitioners, the possibility that an ad-hoc combination may not have the intended effects argues in favor of established formulas that have withstood the test of time.*

[2] *The nomenclature and composition of formulas may vary depending on the historical source, regional and sectarian practice and manufacturere in the case of commercial preparations.*

interactions between component herbs may produce desirable modification of properties, augmenting the beneficial effects and counteracting unwanted effects associated with single herbs; or result in new, synergistic actions. Combination thus has a greater therapeutic effect and greater safety than each ingredient alone.

While an established formula is made up of substances in specified proportions, the ratio as well as the content is ultimately to be adjusted on an individual basis. The use of modern extract preparations instead of traditional decoctions severely limits this flexibility, as will be explained later in detail.

An oft-cited example using ephedra serves to illustrate how combination can achieve different, even opposing actions.(4)

ephedra + cinnamon	diaphoretic
ephedra + gypsum	checks sweating
ephedra + apricot kernel	settles cough (antitussive), calms dyspnea (anti-asthmatic)
ephedra + atractylodes	disinhibits urine (diuretic)

Apparently, particular principles in ephedra are either potentiated or inhibited depending on the nature of the companion herb.

The mechanisms of these interactions are unknown for the most part. Conventional procedures that apply to Western drug evaluation are inadequate for complex incompletely characterized mixtures. Chemical interactions between the compounds of the mixture occur during decoction. Following oral administration, a myriad of molecular encounters occur, in which compounds and their metabolites interact with each other and with the systems of the body during the various stages of absorption, distribution, metabolism, and excretion. In view of such complexity and the limitations of the usual methodology, it is perhaps not surprising that most of Kampo research has been narrowly confined to the study of "active principles." Yet the essential strategy and significance of Kampo medicine as a therapeutic system is to be found in the totality of the formula.

Only recently have some researchers begun to focus on the underlying raison d'etre of Kampo herbal formulations. Some representative discoveries and the hypotheses substantiated by them are cited below.(5,6)

Hypothesis 1: Decocting herbs together affects the amount extracted into solution and thus the bioavailability of their respective ingredients.

For example, the amount of glycyrrhizin in a decoction of licorice root decreased by 53% upon the addition of ephedra, while the ephedrine extracted into a decoction of ephedra is increased by the addition of licorice.

Another experiment was conducted on a formula that has been used for 2000 years in the treatment of asthma. It is composed of four ingredients: ephedra, apricot kernel, licorice, and gypsum.[2] It was observed that the decoction of the mixture of the four substances, at the ratio specified in the classics, had a stronger and-longer-lasting effect[3] than the mixture of separate decoctions of each component,

---

[2] *Ephedra, Apricot Kernel, Licorice, and Gypsum Decoction.*
[3] *Defined by the ED50 of antitussive action in guinea pigs.*

also at the same ratio. The chief difference in chemical composition between the two was that the former contained more ephedrine. This suggests that the presence of the other ingredients enabled more ephedrine to be extracted during decoction.

Hypothesis 2: Each herb in the formula contributes to the overall clinical benefit of that formula.

One line of inquiry attempts to find out whether the original formula prepared by decocting the N ingredient herbs together as instructed in the classics is more efficacious than decoctions of each of the possible combinations of the ingredients, taken 1, 2,..., N-1 at a time. This genre of experiment requires $2^N - 1$ number of decoctions. So far, only simple formulas have been investigated this way. When the above formula for asthma was analyzed, the original formula was found to be the most efficacious in the duration of antitussive effect and second in potency[4] only to the decoction of ephedra alone.

Another line of inquiry makes use of a series of so-called "one-omitted" decoctions, in which one herb is omitted in turn from the original formula. Presumably, if a one-omitted decoction is less effective than the complete formulation, then the omitted herb could be concluded to contribute to the overall effect. When a 9-component remedy[5] was studied in this manner with respect to its anticonvulsant effects, it was found that the complete formula showed the strongest activity[6], and with the exception of *Zingiberis Rhizoma* (ginger root), all herbs make a significant contribution to the anticonvulsant effect. *Zingiberis* is known to reduce the adverse effects of other herbs in the formula, a property which must be assessed with a different experimental protocol.

Hypothesis 3: Not only the presence of an herb, but also its proper proportion relative to the other components, determines the effects of a formula.

In a revealing experiment, three formulas, each with a distinct clinical indication, but differing in composition only in the amount of peony root (0g, 4.0g. and 6.0g. respectively), were investigated with respect to the serum levels of glycyrrhetic acid (derives from licorice root in the formulas) they produced following oral administration.[7] Each produced a distinct serum profile of glycyrrhetic acid with a different maximum and rate of decline. The preparation containing 6.0g. of peony produced the highest maximum level which then dropped off most rapidly. The preparation containing 4.0g. of peony produced the lowest maximum which decreased more gradually. The remaining preparation, containing no peony, produced an intermediate peak that decreased most slowly of all.

The results from these experiments tend to support the empirical axiom that ingredients in a formula act together to produce therapeutic effects not attributable to single herbs or isolated principles.

---

[4] *Ibid.*

[5] *Minor Bupleurum Decoction combined with Cinnamon Twig Decoction Plus Peony.*

[6] *Defined by depression of seizures caused by four different methods in animals.*

[7] *The three formulas were Cinnamon Twig Decoction Minus Peony, Cinnamon Twig Decoction (4.0g peony), and Cinnamon Twig Decoction Plus Peony (6.0g peony).*

C. Normalizing and health-building actions of kampo medicines

Many substances and formulas used in Kampo are recommended for diametrically opposed conditions: hypertension/hypotension, amenorrhea/menorrhagia, depression/excitability, polyuria/oliguria, hypersomnia/hyposomnia, etc. The actions of these remedies appear to be state-dependent: They normalize a function rather than always affect it in the same manner. This understandably invites skepticism in the West, where the current pharmacological paradigm conceives of drugs as invariably exerting a single defined effect, and the methodology of drug development accordingly produces such unidirectional agents.

Empirical use and a growing body of experimental data also show that a number of traditional remedies have general health-building therapeutic effects. They improve mood, mental performance, sleep, appetite, and digestion, and increase vitality and nonspecific resistance, without producing physiological dependence. Again, there is nothing comparable in modern drugs, which tend to erode the state of health when used chronically.

Such normalizing and health-enhancing remedies might be said to have adaptogenic activities. "Adaptogen," a term relatively new and unfamiliar to Western biomedicine, was proposed by Brehkman in 1958 to refer to any nontoxic substance that increases resistance against a wide spectrum of stresses, and which tends to restore physiological norms regardless of the direction of pathological change.(7) That is, an adaptogen raises the capacity of the organism to adapt and enhances resistance to disease. The alternative term "harmony remedy" has also been coined, to emphasize the fact that such substances act by maintaining or restoring homeostasis.(8)

It has been postulated that adaptogens or harmony remedies are capable of modulating a disease process because they are a balanced mixture of chemicals. The body would utilize the components it needs to reinstate homeostasis.(9) Another hypothesis maintains that the remedies contain specific compounds that elicit homeostasis by tuning the hormonal control systems of the body.(8)

The attributes of an adaptogen appear to describe many of the substances in Chinese materia medica that are classified as "superior" medicines. Superior medicines are those substances that are traditionally considered to be mild and harmless, and which increase vitality, prevent senility, and prolong life with continuous use. Substances in this class are often combined in a formula with other ingredients, classified as "medium" or "inferior" according to their degree of toxicity, and having stronger, more defined effects and counter specific disorders. As has been observed, this scheme would place the bulk of modern drugs in the "inferior" category, and sharply highlights the divergent emphasis between biomedicine, which values powerful curative drugs that are intrinsically toxic, and the Chinese medical tradition, which values adjustive and restorative remedies that foster health.(8)

The harmony remedies can be applied in fatigue, weakness, and susceptibility to disease, which are common complaints in the elderly, the convalescent, and those who are weakened by stress. They are certainly beneficial in the peri-menopause, a period of hormonal and psychosocial stress.

The worldwide epidemic of AIDS has deepened our appreciation of the importance of a healthy immune system. There is growing awareness that it is irrational, belated, and costly to devise treatment only after there has been extensive damage. In the face of the unpredictability of disease, the promotion of health itself is crucial. The harmony remedies would be a valuable addition to health-building measures in our stress-ridden society. They, and more importantly, the concepts of health maintenance of the tradition that spawned them, merit candid and scrupulous appraisal in the West.

References for Chapter 3

(1) Weil, Andrew. *Health and Healing.* ch. 9, pp. 103-105. Boston: Houghton Mifflin Co., 1988.

(2) *Ibid.*, p. 110.

(3) Lander, L. *Defective Medicine.* p. 27. New York: Farrar, Straus, Giroux, 1978.

(4) Kuwagi, Takahide. *Ekisuzai ni Yoru Kampō Shinryō Handobukku (Handbook of Kampo Examination and Treatment with Extract Preparations).* pp. 41-42. Tokyo: Sōgensha, 1983.

(5) Hosoya, Eikichi. "Scientific Reevaluation of Kampo Formulas using Modern Technology." In Hosoya, Eikichi, Y. Yamamura. "Recent Advances in the Pharmacology of Kampo (Japanese Herbal) Medicines." *Excerpta Medica,* 1988.

(6) Terasawa, Katsutoshi. "The Significance of the Combined Preparations Used in Kampo Medicine." In Hosoya, Eikichi, Y. Yamamura. "Recent Advances in the Pharmacology of Kampo (Japanese Herbal) Medicines." *Excerpta Medica,* 1988.

(7) Farnsworth, N.R. *et al.* "Siberian Ginseng (Eleutherococcus senticosus): Current Status as an Adaptogen." *Economic and Medicinal Plant Research.* vol.1, Chapter 5. Academic Press, 1985.

(8) Fulder, Stephen. *The Tao of Medicine.* Rutland, VT: Healing Arts Press, 2nd. edition, 1990.

(9) Duke, James. *Ginseng: A Concise Handbook.* Reference Publications, Inc., 1989, p.119.

Chapter 4
Kampo as a Complement to Biomedicine

General interest in Kampo medicine has been rising steadily since World War II. Far from a transient fad, it appears to have earned a stable place in modern Japanese health care.

An epidemiological transition has contributed to the resurgence of Kampo medicine. Incidence of infectious diseases has declined. In place of maladies that take a swift toll on life, chronic diseases that affect the entire body during their slow progression have become the major causes of morbidity and mortality. At the same time, with the increase in average life span, health care needs of the elderly have reached unprecedented proportions. Comorbidity (the coexistence of multiple chronic conditions) is common in older populations. As never before in history, the typical patient is one who harbors many diseases, each of which is not fatal in the near term.

For such patients, therapeutic goals must extend beyond the primary aim of prolonging survival to embrace an improvement in wellbeing and the patient's ability to function; in other words, considerations of quality of life. Thus individual differences between patients become more pertinent relative to the features common to particular chronic ailments.

Hand in hand with the changes in disease and demographic profile, increasing recognition of the inability of modern biomedicine to meet these new challenges has helped to propel Kampo and other alternative systems to the forefront of consideration. Indictments against modern medicine are many, ranging from its fragmented approach with a loss of emphasis on the whole human being, to the creation of iatrogenic problems by the often unwise use of its arsenal of powerful drugs and invasive technology. Such criticisms reflect the state of impasse that modern medicine has reached in its relations with patients, and are best understood as part of a social reassessment of scientific-technological culture.

I. Fields of applications

Kampo may be applied in almost all conditions. Today, however, it is little relied upon in disorders that normally require surgery; and rarely, if ever used in emergency, life-threatening situations. Dominance of the biomedical system tends to relegate it to an adjunct status, so that it is usually not considered as an option where relatively effective modern treatment exists.

From a Western standpoint, the remedies of the greatest interest are those that potentially cover the deficiencies of modern treatments. Generally, these tend to be remedies for functional or chronic disorders. This does not mean that Kampo is not useful in acute or organic disorders. Used in the beginning stage of a cold, it can quickly effect a cure. Kampo treatment is also effective in acute gastritis or enteritis, and has been known to obviate the need for surgery in cases of appendicitis or hernia.

General categories of problems that often respond better to Kampo therapy than conventional medicine are listed below. They overlap to some extent, being categories designed for convenience of presentation.

A. Functional disorders

Cases without significant organic changes, where subjective complaints cannot be correlated with laboratory findings, are particularly suitable for Kampo therapy. In modern medicine, they are variously referred to as nonspecific complaints, functional disturbances, dysfunction of the autonomic nervous system, or psychosomatic disorders. General malaise, lack of energy, or excessive fatigue can also fit this category.

B. Disorders related to the immune system

Deficiency of the immune system, viral infections, allergies, autoimmune disorders, cancers, and other conditions featuring chronic or recurrent infections or chronic inflammations.

C. Unsatisfactory response to modern treatment

Poor response to customarily effective treatment, allergy and other unexpected reactions, or situations where treatment results in quantitative improvement but fails to amelieorate the subjective symptoms.

D. Postoperative recovery, convalescence from debilitating illness

Kampo speeds recovery after surgery, restores proper circulation, and promotes proper healing of wounds. It can be used to treat postoperative complications such as respiratory symptoms, anorexia, GI disturbances, impaired liver functions, urinary problems, adhesions, and fistula formation. Certain formulas may be administered before the operation to increase vitality, help prevent postoperative complications, and accelerate a return to normal activities.

E. Iatrogenic problems

Kampo formulas may be used to counter the harmful effects of otherwise beneficial conventional treatment and help to reduce drug dependence.(1) Some examples are:

§ Kampo therapy can diminish the adverse effects of radiation therapy and anticancer drugs (anemia, leucopenia, anorexia, vomiting, fatigue, immunosuppressive states, etc.); it can also increase the efficacy of anticancer drugs.

§ The incidence and severity of adverse effects associated with corticosteroid drugs depends on the dosage and the length of treatment. Concomitant use of Kampo can have a steroid-sparing effect, leading to dose reduction or even complete withdrawal from steroid treatment.

§ In mild hypertension, conventional drugs that marginally reduce mortality but cause side effects may be replaced with Kampo formulas.

§ One Kampo formula can simultaneously address multiple conditions, thus reducing the risks of polypharmacy.

F. Obstetrics and gynecology

This is traditionally a highly developed specialty of Kampo medicine. Its extensive and richly-nuanced repetoire of remedies may be used to advantage in all problems related to the female reproductive system.

G. Geriatric care

Kampo is beneficial for asthenic or debilitated states. It is suitable for the typical features of geriatric patients: comorbidity, decline in physical and mental functions, impaired immunity and natural healing mechanisms, and susceptibility to drug side effects due to decreased ability to metabolize and excrete drugs.

The benefits of Kampo in the above seemingly diverse categories arise directly from the principal differences between Kampo medicine and biomedicine, as detailed in the last section. We summarize and extend them below.

The first is emphasis on patient perception. Subjective complaints occupy a central position in the diagnostic assessment, which means that it is often possible to attend to incipient problems before they grow into overt manifestations of disease. Whereas Western doctors tend to regard quantitative measurements as the true measure of treatment efficacy, Kampo doctors accord much weight to the patient's perspective and efficacy of treatment is judged above all by the extent to which the symptoms no longer affect a patient's wellbeing and daily activities. Interestingly, clinical experience with Kampo has often shown that amelioration of subjective symptoms can occur without a significant change in objective findings. Where objective improvement is observed, subjective improvement either precedes or parallels it. This highlights the contrast between the Kampo focus on the illness experienced by the patient and the preoccupation of modern medicine with the objective signs of disease.

Emphasis on patient perception is a feature consonant with the growing emphasis on quality of life issues in present-day management of chronic disorders. Kampo can be particularly suitable in clinical situations where quality of life considerations are important, for instance, where treatment is expected to be of marginal benefit with regard to survival, or where therapeutic benefits will likely be offset by effects adverse to the patient's wellbeing.

The holistic interpretation of symptoms is particularly important in chronic illness with systemic involvement or conditions lacking a precise etiology and treatment. In such cases, pattern-thinking is unfettered by boundaries between disease categories and divisions between medical specialties. It can better assemble seemingly unrelated, localized bodily phenomena and account for individual differences. The ability to size up the overall condition of the patient is important in avoiding piecemeal symptomatic treatment and the dangers of polypharmacy.

Finally, the pharmacology of Kampo remedies supports its conceptual and diagnostic orientation. Remedies possess a broad spectrum of actions that address whole cluster of symptoms. Many drugs have a negative impact on the quality of life and can cause poor compliance and withdrawal from therapy. By contrast, Kampo medicines for chronic disorders have mild but progressive actions and low incidence of associated side effects. Therapeutic benefits include immune enhancement, normalization of body functions, and improvement of alertness, mood, memory, and feelings of wellbeing.

II. Cooperation

Despite the radical divergence between Kampo and Western medicine on both conceptual and practical levels, the two modalities are not necessarily incompatible. Indeed, since the avowed objective of medicine is to care for the patient in the best way possible, it would be desirable to unite their respective strengths to create a more comprehensive and humanistic system of prevention and treatment.

How such a combination may be realized in actual clinical practice is suggested to some extent by the type and stage of the condition to be treated. In general, Western management and drugs take precedence in acute infectious or inflammatory diseases, acute flare-ups of chronic conditions, emergencies, and malignancies. Kampo can then be utilized as maintenance therapy to improve chronic disorders, to help prevent recurrences, and to assist postoperative recovery. Where Western management is beneficial but produces substantial side effects or fails to alleviate subjective symptoms, Kampo can be used adjunctively to reduce toxicities and complications, and to reinforce the efficacy of modern therapy. Kampo may be the principal therapy in various functional disorders, in mild to moderate cases of cold-like syndromes, in diseases lacking effective modern treatment (e.g., chronic hepatitis), or in cases of drug intolerance.

These are not ironclad rules. Combination therapy is an on-going research topic, and much remains unknown. Ultimately, the optimum mix depends on individual patient characteristics. For this reason combination therapy is perhaps best managed by the same practitioner, schooled in both systems, who can tailor the treatment regimen based on the patient's condition, response, and progress. Collaboration between a physician and a Kampo practitioner can also result in a personal shaping of the treatment regimen, but would require intimate coordination, mutual comprehension, and respect for each other's craft.

Reference for Chapter 4

(1) Hosoya, Eikichi. "Scientific Reevaluation of Kampo Formulas Using Modern Technology." In Hosoya, Eikichi and Y. Yamamura, eds. "Recent Advances in the Pharmacology of Kampo (Japanese Herbal) Medicines." *Excerpta Medica,* 1988.

PART II

INTRODUCTION TO KAMPO PRACTICE

Chapter 5
Basic Concepts

T his chapter introduces the concept of formula pattern as well as several traditional constructs of pathology useful in the framework of this manual.

I. Formula Pattern *(hōshō)*

Depending on the context, a pattern in Kampo can mean:
- The constellation of a patient's signs and symptoms, either locally or overall
- Information gathered with a particular diagnostic method
- Characteristics of a particular type of pathology
- A cluster of symptoms and signs indicating treatment by a particular formula — a formula pattern

It is this last genre that is accented in Kampo, and is therefore the focus here. In the interest of brevity, the term "pattern" is generally employed without further qualification in the rest of the book, with the understanding that it stands for formula pattern.

Correspondence between formulas and patterns

The core of Kampo practice is based on the concept of a "key-and-lock" relationship between remedies and patterns of signs and symptoms. Each established remedy is coupled with a pattern, which is customarily named after the remedy. For example, the pattern treated by Cinnamon and Poria Pills is called the Cinnamon and Poria Pills pattern, and when this pattern is diagnosed in a patient, Cinnamon and Poria Pills is directly indicated. Because of this pre-established scheme of correspondences, a formula pattern serves double duty in Kampo. It not only functions as a basic unit or category of diagnosis, but also defines the circumstances in which its corresponding formula can be applied. The ultimate significance of a pattern lies in its being a specific treatment warrant.[1]

---

[1] *The term "Shō" which we have loosely translated as pattern, means proof or evidence in everyday use of the word in Japanese, and underscores the fact that when a patterns is diagnosed, it substantiates treatment by its corresponding remedy.*

Pattern as a representation of illness

A pattern in Kampo is in some sense the counterpart of disease in biomedicine. Much as modern physicians diagnose diseases, Kampo physicians diagnose patterns. Both are representations of the patient's illness at a point in time, a distillation of the features of the case from which proper treatment may proceed. But while biomedical disease entities are framed in terms of current understandings of pathoanatomy and pathophysiology, Kampo patterns are clinical and empirical accounts of illness. Typically, a pattern is defined by an enumeration of clinical features, including elements of subjective complaints, history, physical findings, and individual factors (see Part IV for examples). There is minimal explicit consideration of the events underlying the manifestations of illness.

This descriptive approach might be seen as a nosology (classification of disease) based on clinical features, which little depends on models of etiology or pathogenesis.[2] What is more, the direct coupling of pattern (diagnosis) with remedy (specific treatment) in Kampo implies a treatment-specific nosology, where pathologic conditions are differentiated and categorized according to the appropriate means of treatment. This treatment-specific nosology is an abiding legacy of the positivist and result-oriented philosophy of the Classical school. Most Kampo physicians tend to brush by theoretical considerations, asking not so much, "How did this disorder arise and develop?" but straightaway, "What can be used to restore health in a patient with this constellation of signs and symptoms and background factors?" Although the present trend is toward rationalization, by and large, Kampo today is still a clinical medicine emphasizing the direct perception of problems experienced by the patients and solutions for them with few intervening explanatory models.

Content of a pattern

From a modern perspective, many Kampo patterns may appear to be whimsical collections of findings. Seemingly trivial phenomena are often included and sometimes accorded cardinal significance. Partly, this is because a pattern arises from a clinical rather than an etiological or anatomical view of illness. Also, since the concerns and presuppositions of physicians in the past often bear little resemblance to current understandings, the line between what counts as noise and what counts as information was drawn differently.

It is instructive to compare a pattern with a syndrome. The latter is a cluster of signs and symptoms that characterizes a particular disorder. They are similar in that both consist of a collection of clinical features. However, a pattern often contains information that, from a modern perspective, is more aptly called predisposing or contributing factors, susceptibilities, or constitutional tendencies, rather than signs or symptoms. One might also refer to such information collectively as responder characteristics (the traits of an individual who will respond favorably to a medication), since a pattern also functions as a set of indications for its corresponding formula.

---

[2] *Such clinical nosologies still survive in areas of medicine where theory does not furnish effective explanations of clinical phenomena. A salient example is the nosology developed by the American Psychiatric Association in its Diagnostic and Statistical Manual of Mental Disorders (DSM-III).*

Not all patterns include detailed responder characteristics. Some consist mostly or exclusively of signs and symptoms, and bear more similarity to syndromes or indications for drugs. This can be the case when the corresponding formula is created largely for the purpose of symptom relief, or the nature of the remedy may be such that it is applicable in a wide range of patient types.

As is true for a syndrome, not all elements in a pattern carry the same diagnostic weight. A distinction is made between major and minor features, or equivalently from the therapeutic standpoint, major and minor indications for its corresponding formula. The former are the essential elements of the pattern, and are generally required in its identification. The latter are often but not necessarily present. They generally have accessory importance in making the diagnosis. One might think of the major features as setting the tenor of the pattern, and the minor ones as being its more variable or transitory components.

Pattern diagnosis and the dynamic nature of illness

A pattern is a treatment-oriented summary of the patient's illness (or a subset of it) at a point in time. Changes in the clinical presentation with time must be reflected in the pattern used to characterize it. This reformulation of pattern diagnosis is analogous to the reformulation of biomedical diagnosis to account for the emergence and progression of disease processes. However, because it tracks overall changes in symptoms and signs as well as constitutional factors, pattern diagnosis is often more labile than biomedical diagnosis, which typically remains the same in chronic disorders.

Pattern diagnosis and the dynamic nature of medicine

The biomedical cooptation of Kampo in Japan has created impetus to update traditional definitions of patterns with modern medical knowledge and diagnostic techniques. These efforts are expected to produce supplementary quantitative criteria for the application of traditional remedies and, as has been demonstrated for several formulas, even lead to entirely new areas of application.

II. Selected Concepts of Pathology

Although the prevailing mode of practice centers on direct pattern-formula correspondence, a number of basic concepts of pathology are often used to guide clinical decisions. They have survived the vicissitudes of past medical reforms largely because of their utility in characterizing and unifying phenomena, allowing motley clinical findings to be sorted into categories, which can be thought of as subpatterns. As such, they facilitate overall pattern discernment and indicate the pertinence of particular therapeutic agents.

A handful of such fundamental concepts are discussed in the following pages. True to Kampo's practical orientation, the presentation here focuses on signs and symptoms, i.e., the expressions of the pathologies concerned, not their genesis or evolution.[3] Parallels are drawn with biomedical concepts, and modern terminology is used wherever possible. Readers interested in a systematic exposition of

---

[3] Recall that a sign or a symptom has no absolute meaning in Kampo but assumes particular significance in the light of the entire pattern. Exclusive association should not be assumed between a pathology and the signs or symptoms cited in conjunction with it.

Oriental medicine promoted in contemporary China can turn to a text such as *Fundamentals of Chinese Medicine* by Wiseman and Ellis (see Bibliography).

A. Constitutional State *(taishitsu)*

One of the objects of diagnosis is to assess a set of individual factors, which we shall refer to as "constitutional state." This rubric stands for the general characteristics of body structure, diatheses (predispositions), degree of vitality, and capacity to withstand untoward circumstances – factors that collectively form the ground matrix of a pattern of imbalance.

Constitutional state cannot be evaluated in any absolute sense, but only qualitatively. We will employ the terms "sthenia" (from Greek sthenos, strength) and "asthenia" (a-, without + sthenos, strength) to designate the two poles of a continuum between a robust state and a frail (or adynamic) state.[4]

Typical attributes of these opposites are summarized in the table on the following page.[5] As suggested by the table, constitutional state is not one-dimensional, but a composite indication of reserve ("supply" of mental and physical vigor) and resistance, derived from a comprehensive evaluation of multiple traits. Neither is it static. While some attributes, such as type of physique, are relatively stable, others can fluctuate over the course of illness and over the life cycle. A Tarzan can be enfeebled by chronic infection, while a Popeye can build up hardiness and resistance through proper diet and exercise.

Among the traits listed in the table, the state of the abdominal wall has particular significance in the assessment of constitutional state. See "Abdominal Strength," p. 59 for a discussion.

For convenience, a five-level ordinal scale is adopted throughout the book to codify constitutional state:

> 5 = sthenic; having the typical attributes of sthenia
>
> 4 = somewhat sthenic; some attributes of sthenia or a preponderance of sthenic over asthenic attributes
>
> 3 = intermediate; tending neither to sthenia nor asthenia
>
> 2 = somewhat asthenic; some attributes of asthenia or a preponderance of asthenic over sthenic attributes
>
> 1 = asthenic; having the typical attributes of asthenia

This scale is admittedly rough and simplistic. It suffices nonetheless, for the value of constitutional state in Kampo diagnosis is general orientation of the therapeutic method.

---

[4] *The common meaning of the Kampo terms "kyo" and "jitsu," which we have translated as asthenia and sthenia, differ from their counterparts in Chinese medicine. In Chinese, kyo means vacuity, and denotes functional and substantive insufficiency or depletion. Jitsu means repletion, and signifies the strength of pathogen or abundance of pathological products. These terms are used to designate the type of pathology, not the constitutional state. The Kampo usage probably grew out of the observation that repletion-type pathology is usually associated with sthenic persons, and vacuity-type pathology with asthenic persons.*

[5] *Based on works by Kazuo Tatsuno, as cited by H. Nishiyama in Kampō Igaku no Kiso to Shinryō (Principles and Practice of Kampo Medicine).*

Table One	Sthenia and Asthenia: Comparison of Attributes	

	STHENIA	ASTHENIA
Body type	thickset or athletic	thin, ptotic
	robust even if overweight	flaccid obesity if overweight
Skin	good nutritional status	poor nutritional status
	has luster and turgor	lack of luster and turgor
Muscle	well-developed	poorly developed
	good tone and elasticity	poor tone and elasticity
	thick, elastic abdominal wall	thin, soft abdominal wall
Digestive system	good digestive function	poor digestive function
	no adverse effects from skipping a meal	feels weak on an empty stomach
		lethargy after eating
	prefers/tolerates cold foods and drinks	tendency toward digestive upsets
		from cold food and drinks
	tendency toward constipation	tendency toward diarrhea or atonic
		constipation
	constipation quickly produces discomfort	no bowel movement for several days
		does not produce significant discomfort
	purging brings about relief	susceptible to adverse GI effects of
		laxative and other drugs
Regulation of body temperature	tolerant of summer heat and winter cold	prone to exhaustion from summer heat
		cold sensitivity
		tendency toward excess perspiration
Activity	vigorous movement	slow-moving
		disinclined to physical movement
	has stamina, recovers quickly from fatigue	tires easily, lingering fatigue
Attitude	positive, assertive	negative, passive
Voice	loud, energetic	soft, thin, faint
Typical pathology	hyper-tonus, hyper-reaction,	hypo-tonus, hypo-reaction,
	accumulation, excess	leakage, insufficiency

Sthenic patients tend to react vigorously or energetically to disease, exhibiting an elevated state of physiological functions. They are more susceptible to the diseases of excess (hypertension, hyperlipidemia, gout, etc.), and generally respond well to treatment that stresses "attack" or "drainage," i.e., direct, active attempts to rid the body of pathogens or pathological products. Formulas with more drastic effects may be employed. By contrast, asthenic patients typically show a weak healing response. They tend to experience gastrointestinal side effects from pharmacotherapy. Accordingly, the emphasis of treatment is on "supplementation," using substances that nourish, improve the digestive function, support immunity, and build vitality. Formulas with milder, progressive effects are usually more suitable.

To summarize, a correspondence could be set up between the general therapeutic character of a remedy and the range of constitutional states in which the remedy is usually applicable. Evaluation of the patient's constitutional state is thus a preliminary step in selecting the proper remedy.

Note that, depending on the primary features of the pattern, this kind of correspondence can be more a rule of safety than of effectiveness. For example, to treat acute inflammation in an asthenic patient, a strong sthenically-oriented remedy may be necessary. But it is generally true that more drastic remedies are more likely to precipitate adverse reactions in asthenic patients, while supplementing remedies are more likely to be either ineffective or harmful in sthenic patients, especially in conditions requiring long-term treatment. By adhering to this correspondence, novices will less likely commit serious mistakes.

B. Cold and Heat *(kan netsu)*

In Kampo, the rubrics "cold" and "heat" not only describe local or systemic temperature or heat production, but also stand for physiological over- or under-activity as well as the signs and symptoms related to these polar states. This distinction helps to guide the selection substances and remedies, as cooling agents are used for heat and warming agents are used for cold.

A mix of cold and heat signs is commonly encountered in clinical practice. A pertinent example is vasomotor instability in the perimenopause where patients present with both hot flushes and cold extremities, and may be intolerant to both heat and cold (see p. 42, "Upper body heat and lower body cold").

We shall refer to chronic lack of body warmth as "coldness syndrome." This is discussed more extensively below.

Typical attributes of cold and heat are listed in the following table. They overlap with those listed under sthenia and asthenia, since there tends to be an association between asthenia and cold, and sthenia and heat.

Table Two   Cold and Heat: Comparison of Attributes

COLD	HEAT
pallor	ruddy complexion
subjective sensations of cold	subjective sensations of heat
decreased blood flow	hyperemia / inflammation
cold sensitivity	heat sensitivity
symptoms worsened by cold & relieved by warming	symptoms worsened by heat & relieved by cooling
no thirst (moist mouth),	thirst with desire for cold drinks;
or thirst with desire for warm drinks	bitter taste in the mouth, halitosis
thin, clear secretions/excretions:	thick, sticky, or colored secretions/excretions:
long micturition with light-colored urine	dark-colored urine
thin, copious vaginal discharge	thick, scant vaginal discharge
watery diarrhea	dry hard stools
desire for quietude, sluggishness	irritability, agitation, restlessness, insomnia

C. Coldness Syndrome *(hieshō)*[6]

Coldness syndrome is characterized by chronic sensations of coldness, which can be systemic or local, affecting one to multiple parts of the body – most commonly the extremities and the lower torso. Cold sensitivity is likely to be an accompanying feature.

The degree of chilliness varies from patient to patient, and from site to site in the same patient. In severe cases, the patient cannot tolerate fans or air conditioning even on a hot summer day, and must always insulate the affected part.

The affected part may not feel cold to others. It may be a purely subjective phenomenon that cannot be verified by measurement of skin temperature. However, subjective complaints of coldness usually agree with objective observation. Patients complaining of cold feet almost always have feet that are cold to the touch.

Incidence

Coldness syndrome tends to be more prevalent and severe in those living in colder regions. But their occurrence is not restricted to the winter season or the northern climes.

Asthenic individuals are more susceptible. Women are predominantly affected, especially those in middle age and perimenopausal years. Hormonal and anatomical differences are believed to contribute to this bias. In men, the elderly constitute the majority of patients.

Significance

The likes of cold hands and feet may seem a trivial problem requiring only more layers of clothing. They are given attention in Kampo because, first of all, they may be distressful to the patient, and Kampo practitioners are above all heedful of the patient's subjective wellbeing. Second, they have diagnostic value in the determination of the nature of imbalance, and therefore the proper therapy. Sometimes, the location and degree of cold by themselves are necessary and sufficient indication for a particular remedy.

Not least, even if not serious in itself, coldness syndrome is thought to contribute to the pathogenesis of a host of disorders, or to their perpetuation. Longstanding coldness syndrome tends to be observed in conjunction with circulatory, gastrointestinal, neuroendocrine, and metabolic disorders. But it can be associated with disturbances in virtually all body systems.

Special relevance to gynecology

Coldness syndrome is observed in a great many women with menstrual disorders, pelvic congestion syndrome, climacteric disturbances, or nonspecific complaints. It has been estimated that four times as many women with menstrual disorders are affected as those without.

---

[6] *This discussion is based on the Japanese experience. While its pertinence remains to be demonstrated conclusively in the West, Chinese herbalists and acupuncturists do regularly observe and treat coldness syndrome in the United States.*

An anatomical explanation has been advanced to account for the greater incidence of coldness syndrome in women. Compared to men, women have more subcutaneous fat deposit in the buttocks and the lower abdomen, which protects and insulates the reproductive organs sandwiched in between. The nature of the fat layer is such that once warmed, it does not cool easily; conversely, once cooled, it does not warm up easily. When the lower body (including the lower extremities) becomes chilled, low-temperature blood circulates back to the abdomen from the lower extremities. This blood chills the pelvis, including the fat layer, which then no longer keeps the reproductive organs warm, and indeed, tends to retard the return of warmth. Suboptimal temperature can in turn engender other abnormalities that precipitate a host of women's disorders.

Western parallels

Coldness syndrome is so prosaic in the fabric of Japanese reality that many Japanese are surprised by the absence of an exact translation in English. Others express disbelief that Occidentals, whom they imagine to be robust carnivores, can have problems with cold hands and feet.

Coldness syndrome does have a rough counterpart in Western herbal tradition, where cold extremities, susceptibility to chilblains, etc. are summarily referred to as poor circulation. Herbalists past and present treat manifestations of poor circulation with warming and circulatory stimulant herbs such as ginger and cayenne.

In conventional medicine, coldness syndrome is in general not regarded as an illness requiring treatment, unless associated with well-defined disease entities. These include hypothyroidism, Raynaud's phenomenon, and occlusive vascular disorders, as well as chilblains.

Coldness syndrome can often be considered in terms of peripheral circulatory insufficiency. One probable mechanism is capillary constriction and reduction of blood flow, caused by functional disturbances of the autonomic nervous system involving the vasomotor component. But this fails to describe purely subjective coldness sensations. It has been speculated that the perception of surface temperature stimulus is influenced in an as yet unknown way by changes in core body temperature.

Etiologic factors

Excessive exposure to cold and/or dampness in the environment, prevalence of air-conditioning, overconsumption of cold foods and drinks, sedentary habits, and occupations requiring long periods of standing are external and lifestyle factors that contribute to the genesis of coldness syndrome.

Endogenous factors are not clearly understood in modern pathophysiological terms.

Diagnosis

Usually, diagnosis is based on the subjective sensations and complaints of the patient. In Japan, where coldness syndrome is a household concept, patients would often volunteer the information and sometimes seek treatment solely on account of it. In the West, patients would rarely mention it during medical history intake, let alone go to a doctor for treatment. Clinicians in the West should therefore rely more on observation, palpation, and pointed inquiry to diagnose this condition.

The extremities, abdomen, and back should be palpated to see if they are cold to the touch. This can be carried out easily while performing abdominal palpation (Chapter 7). Questions can be asked at the same time, to learn whether the patient perceives the cold and is bothered by it, and whether she is sensitive or intolerant to cold.

Other signs culled by general observation and questioning that suggest asthenia, such as thinness, preference for warm food and drink, or tendency toward digestive upsets after eating cold or raw foods may also indicate the presence of coldness syndrome.

Careful investigation is necessary to uncover any possible underlying disease, such as organic disorder of the peripheral artery.

Treatment

In Japan, functional coldness syndrome has been treated variously by vasodilators, hormone therapy (estrogen and androgen), vitamin E supplements, psychotropic drugs, and psychotherapy, all with little success. Kampo medicine is generally acknowledged to be more effective for coldness syndrome. Upwards of 40 different extract preparations are commonly available. As always, choice of remedy must be determined by the overall pattern of imbalance.

D. Headrushes *(nobose)*[7]

The term "headrush" is used in this book to denote the Japanese expression *nobose,* itself rendered by two characters meaning "reverse" or "un-natural," and "up," signifying a contra-normal movement upward. Dictionaries generally translate *nobose* as a rush of blood to the head, or a feverish or excited state.

Nobose refers to an uncomfortable sensation of heat, congestion, or mounting pressure in the upper body, especially in the head, often with visible flushing in the face. The phenomenon occurs episodically and lasts a few minutes or longer.

Headrush includes the phenomenon of hot flush, but is broader in scope. Elsewhere, it has been translated as "flushing up." The expression "headrush" is adopted here because flushing, or turning red, is not necessarily a feature.

---

[7] *Headrush is traditionally included in the category of qi imbalances. The trio of qi, blood, and fluid are said to flow throughout the body and sustain all life activity. Qi imbalances are not discussed as such in this text, which does not cover traditional theories of physiology. For readers familiar with the concept of qi in Chinese medicine, we note that the types of qi imbalances emphasized in Kampo can be grouped under headrushes and neuropsychologic disturbances (nervous tension, anxiety, depression, etc.), while the construct of qi vacuity is often expressed in terms of asthenia and weak digestive function.*

One or more of the following symptoms often accompany headrushes:
- hyperemia (flushing, ocular rubor, etc.)
- headache
- palpitations
- dizziness
- heavy-headedness
- cold extremities, cold lower body
- sweating from the head or upper body
- neck and shoulder stiffness
- tinnitus
- thirst/mouth dryness
- irritability, insomnia

This cluster of symptoms is referred to collectively as *nobose shō,* the "headrush syndrome."[8] Note the overlap with heat symptomatology.

Headrushes can be considered a local sign of heat. In particular, when cold lower body and extremities is a significant part of the headrush syndrome, the term "upper body heat and lower body cold" is customarily used to describe the condition.[9]

Headrush syndrome can be a normal physiologic reaction to certain stressors. However, if it causes distress by being prolonged, severe, or frequent, then it requires treatment. Substances such as cinnamon or coptis are specific for this condition. Therefore, formulas containing these substances are potentially applicable when headrushes figure in the symptom picture.

Modern correlates

Although not a condition identified in modern medicine, the state of autonomic imbalance described by headrush syndrome is common in patients affected by cardiovascular diseases and gynecologic disorders (such as climacteric syndrome, menstrual disorders, fibroids, endometriosis, and pelvic congestion syndrome), as well as the following conditions:
- neuroses
- insomnia
- migraine
- hyperthyroidism
- stomatitis
- constipation
- polycythemia
- febrile disorders
- burn injuries

---

[8] *In Chinese medicine, classical concepts of pathology related to headrush syndrome include:*

qì nì	*qi counterflow*
shàng rè xià hán	*upper body heat and lower body cold*
shàng shí xià xū	*upper body repletion and lower body vacuity*
gān yáng shàng kàng	*ascendant hyperactivity of liver yang*
xīn gān huǒ wàng	*upflaming of heart and liver fire*

[9] *The normal state may be described as "upper body cold and lower body heat," that is, the head is cooler in temperature relative to the feet in a healthy human being. The term "upper body heat and lower body cold," though restricted in this manual to the sense specified in the text (as is usual in Kampo), can potentially refer to other combinations of heat signs in the upper body and cold signs in the lower body.*

As is true for hot flushes, environmental stresses such as crowded rooms or stuffy air can precipitate an episode of headrush syndrome; so may wearing too much clothing, soaking too long in a hot bath, emotional stress, vigorous activities, hot or spicy food and drinks, or excessive intake of caffeine or alcohol. It can also be iatrogenic, occurring as an adverse reaction to pharmacotherapy (including herbal remedies) and acumoxa therapy.

The concept of headrush syndrome ties together seemingly unrelated minor nuisance complaints, and can be useful in the management of these subjective symptoms seen in a multitude of disorders.

E. Blood imbalances *(ketsushō)*

1. Blood stasis *(oketsu)*

Blood stasis is a Kampo concept used to guide the diagnosis and treatment of a plethora of disorders. It is all-important in the field of gynecology, serving to explain wholly or partially many common conditions, including menstrual disorders, endometriosis, dysfunctional bleeding, fibroids, and infertility.

In its most narrow and concrete sense, blood stasis designates blood that is no longer free-flowing and has lost its physiological function; namely, stagnant blood in the vessels (venous congestion, blood clot, thrombus, etc.) or extravasated blood accumulating in surrounding tissues (internal bleeding). Since all physiologic activities depend on proper blood circulation, it is intuitively clear that stagnancy, like a congestion in a drainage pipe, can create all kinds of housekeeping problems for the human body. By extension, blood stasis can also refer to these complications or secondary disorders.[10]

Centered on the modern concept of impaired microcirculation (blood flow within the tiny veins and capillaries), attempts to define the pathology of blood stasis have identified it with several interrelated abnormalities:(1)
 • abnormally high blood density or viscosity
 • defects in the clotting or anti-clotting mechanisms
 • vascular damage or obstruction
 • congestion due to increased flow of blood to the area, reduced drainage of blood from the area, or backpressure in the circulation

These can give rise to secondary changes, such as:
 • insufficient blood supply (e.g., impaired perfusion of organs and tissues due to microthrombus formation)
 • bleeding (e.g., due to abnormal clotting process)
 • lesions (e.g., scarring)
 • systemic or local edema (increased vascular permeability due to congestion)
 • neuroendocrine and other imbalances

These can further derange microvascular blood flow, perpetuating a vicious cycle.

---

[10] *Because of the traditional emphasis on blood stasis and the inter-relatedness of the possible types of blood imbalances, the Kampo concept of blood stasis in its broadest sense can encompass all major pathologies of the blood in traditional Chinese medicine: blood stasis, bleeding, and aspects of blood heat and blood vacuity.*

• **Modern disease entities**

Blood stasis is usually significant in the following conditions:(2)

1. Acute inflammatory disorders, e.g., impact trauma.

2. Chronic inflammatory disorders, e.g., chronic hepatitis, inflammatory bowel disease, rheumatoid arthritis.

3. Pathologic changes of blood and vessels, e.g., varicose veins, hemorrhoids, arteriosclerosis, hyperlipidemia, purpura, hyperviscosity syndrome, disseminated intravascular coagulation.

4. Gynecologic disorders, e.g., menstrual disorders, fibroids, infertility, complications of abortion, postpartum disorders.

Some features of blood stasis are commonly detected in numerous other chronic illnesses.

• **Diagnosis** (1,3)

Blood stasis (BS) can present with a broad spectrum of symptoms and signs depending on the etiology, secondary changes, and the part of the body affected. As yet, there is no uniform standard for the assessment of blood stasis. Below is a proposed set of diagnostic criteria:

MAJOR INDICATIONS

• *Blood stasis abdominal signs*
These abdominal signs (see p. 66) by themselves are sufficient to establish a diagnosis of BS. They can be absent in acute injuries, but are always present in endogenous or chronic cases. They often constitute the first and only indication of impaired circulation in the pre-disease stage.

• *Abnormal dark red, purple, bluish, or blackish coloration*
This is one of the hallmarks of BS. Such colors may be visible in the complexion; the lips, tongue, gums, and linings of the mouth; circles under the eyes; the nail beds; and spots of skin discoloration. They may also be observed in connection with bleeding, as in purpuric spots, blood that contains dark clots, or black tarry feces caused by bleeding in the upper gastrointestinal tract.

• *Pain of fixed location*
Tenderness to pressure may be a feature, and the pain may worsen at night. Tumorous growth can sometimes be detected at the painful site.

• *Vascular abnormalities*
These include capillary dilatation (examples are visible network of capillaries in the palms or legs, and spider nevi on the upper body), dilatation or tortuous appearance of veins (under the tongue, in the legs), and narrowing or blockage of blood vessels.

• *Pathologic tissue growth*
This includes tumors, hyperplasia, or hypertrophy of organs or tissues.

• *Bleeding, tendency to bleed or develop bruises*

OTHER INDICATIONS

   • *Menstrual disorders, or other gynecologic disorders and obstetric complications.*[11]

   • *Dryness of skin and mucous membranes*
   Dry rough lusterless skin, thickening and scaling of skin, dry chapped lips, and mouth dryness are also associated with BS.

   • *Psychologic symptoms*
   Emotional instability, anxiety, depression, mania, insomnia, impaired memory.

   • *Sensory disturbances (such as numbness and tingling), paralysis*

   • *Heat sensations*
   In conjunction with other signs, flushing, local sensation of heat (such as in the hands or feet), feverish sensation, or upper body heat and lower body cold can indicate BS).

The above indications are summarized in Table 3 along with a set of modern diagnostic findings associated with blood stasis.

Table 3

DIAGNOSIS OF BLOOD STASIS
Major indications:
BS abdominal signs Dark red, purple, blue or black coloration Pain of fixed location Vascular abnormalities Pathologic tissue growth Bleeding, tendency to bleed or develop bruises
Other indications:
Menstrual disorders Dryness of skin and mucous membranes Psychologic symptoms Numbness, tingling, paralysis Heat sensations
Modern diagnostic findings
Impaired microvascular blood flow Abnormality in blood rheology Increased platelet aggregation Increased blood viscosity Presence of thrombus Abnormality in the pelvis and lumbar vertebrae

---

[11] *In men, urinary symptoms related to prostatic problems.*

Among the modern techniques that can be used to detect BS, X-rays of the pelvis may possibly furnish the earliest objective evidence of abnormality.(4) Organs and soft tissues are not the only structures to be affected by impaired blood flow. The bones also contain networks of blood vessels and depend on proper circulation for nutrition, growth, and repair. Deformation, atrophy, hardening, osteoporosis, etc. can arise from BS. X-rays of the pelvis and lumbar spine can reveal such changes in the lower lumbar vertebrae, sacrum, ilium, sacroiliac joint, ischium, pubis, and pubic symphysis.(5)

One or more positive test result is diagnostic of BS, even if no definite disease process can be identified. However, laboratory evidence is unlikely in the absence of BS abdominal signs or some other clinical indications. Tests are therefore more for the purpose of confirming the diagnosis. From a Western perspective, test results help to establish a precise medical diagnosis, and are objective measures useful in monitoring the course of BS disorders.(6)

2. Blood vacuity *(kekkyo)*[12]

Blood vacuity refers to the pattern of signs postulated to result from insufficiency of blood and/or of its nourishing function. It is broader in scope than anemia, defined to be a quantitative shortage of red blood cells, hemoglobin, or both. A patient can manifest blood vacuity without clearly measurable abnormality in blood composition or volume.

Blood vacuity is characterized by such signs as pallor (of complexion, tongue, nails), poor nutritional status (dry, lusterless, rough, or chapped skin; dry lifeless hair or excessive hair loss; brittle nails), eye fatigue or blurred vision, dizziness, and palpitations. Other symptoms include skeletal muscle spasms (such as cramps in the calves), sensory disturbances such as numbness in the extremities, psychologic changes such as reduced concentration and sleep disturbances, scanty or irregular menstruation, or light-colored menses.

• Modern disease entities

Other than in various forms of anemia, blood vacuity is often diagnosed in bleeding disorders, hypomenorrhea, skin disorders such as eczema and pruritis senilis, inflammatory bowel disease, neuropathy associated with diabetes mellitus, rheumatoid arthritis, chronic hepatitis, and heart failure.

F. Fluid imbalances *(suishō, suidoku)*

Perspiration

The state of perspiration can have major diagnostic significance in Kampo. The presence or absence of perspiration is especially important in staging acute febrile diseases, and may be a decisive factor in choosing one remedy over another.

---

[12] *The pathology of blood vacuity is often subsumed under blood stasis in the Classical tradition of Kampo. Until the recent intensification of efforts to adopt TCM theory, it was commonly conceptualized as asthenic-type or yin-type blood stasis with signs suggestive of anemia.*

Apart from febrile diseases and psychological stress, unusual sweating is generally associated with the following conditions:

• debilitated state from exhaustion, serious illness, or hemorrhage

• constitutional asthenia characterized by deficient immune function

• abnormality in the water balance (in conjunction with signs such as changes in urinary output, thirst, or edema)

• imbalance of the autonomic nervous system (e.g., menopausal vasomotor instability)

Two technical terms regarding perspiration are used in this book. Spontaneous sweating means unusual or excessive sweating not produced by diaphoretics. Night sweating refers to spontaneous sweating during sleep. Tendency to spontaneous sweating, day or night, is principally observed in asthenic patterns.

Edema

Edema may be a consequence of kidney, heart, liver, or other diseases that generally require medical attention. Although Kampo therapy can be beneficial in such cases, it should in principle be conducted as an adjunct alongside modern treatment.

In women, edema tends to be associated with hormonal imbalance. In general, it is detectable as weight gain, and can cause symptoms such as bloated abdomen, swollen breasts, swollen extremities, puffy face, sense of heaviness or sluggishness in the lower body, paresthesia of the hands and feet, and fibrositis. More acute symptoms can arise from localized water retention. Examples include headache, dizziness (from increased fluid in the labyrinth), eye pain, and joint pain and stiffness. Kampo treatment can be very effective for such fluid retention states seen in premenstrual syndrome and menopause.

Fluid imbalances

Abnormal sweating and edema can be considered subsets of a class of conditions termed fluid imbalances in Kampo, which may be defined as any pathological distribution, discharge (secretion, excretion, exudation), or stagnation of a bodily fluid or semifluid other than blood.[13] It is a concept in age-old humoral pathology that unites phenomena considered disparate from the viewpoint of modern medicine.

Manifestations of fluid imbalances are legion. Rather than presenting a desultory "laundry list" of symptoms, we have attempted to group representative ones by shared characteristics:

• Any abnormality in fluids elaborated and released by the body, i.e., sweat, saliva, tears, nasal discharge, urine, vaginal discharge; manifests as abnormality in perspiration, thirst, etc.

• Obstruction of the respiratory passages, as by sputum or pleural exudate, causing congestion, coughing, dyspnea, etc.

---

13 *The fluid imbalances in Kampo correspond to the disorders of the fluids in Chinese medicine.*

• GI disturbances, such as epigastric discomfort, poor appetite, substernal splashing sound (p. 64), abdominal rumbling, nausea and vomiting, and diarrhea, which are considered to result from stagnation of stomach secretion and partially digested food particles.

• Symptoms that can derive from local or generalized water retention as discussed above; or more generally, from circulatory disturbances: bloatedness, headache, dizziness, visible swelling, numbness and tingling, palpitations, etc. General sites of water accumulation and examples of associated symptoms are:

• in tissues or body cavities   puffiness, swelling
• in the muscle   sense of heaviness, stiffness, laborious movement
• beneath the scalp   heavy-headedness, bag-over-the-head sensation
• inside the cranium   dizziness, susceptibility to motion sickness
• compressing blood vessels or nerves   numbness and tingling, dull pain, muscle spasm

As is evident from the above enumeration, the symptomatology of fluid imbalance encompasses diverse disorders, from bronchitis, asthma, and gastritis, to rheumatism, cystitis, kidney, and heart diseases. They have one common denominator: the deviation of one or more bodily fluids (semifluids) from their normal ranges.[14]

Fluid stagnation and its clinical manifestations is the aspect of fluid imbalance traditionally emphasized in Kampo, apparently on account of its epidemiologic importance over other types of fluid imbalance in Japan.[15] Conditions characterized by fluid stagnation are likely to be associated with cold sensitivity, and tend to worsen with exposure to cold or damp in the environment.

Fluid imbalance provides a conceptual underpinning for the astounding scope of applications of certain Kampo remedies. Where pertinent, we will invoke this idea to illuminate the interconnection between symptoms and similarity between different diseases.

G. Weak Gastrointestinal Function *(ichō kyojaku)*[16]

In perimenopausal women, aging-related functional decline of the GI tract in combination with poor nutrition can easily set the stage for fatigue, depression, osteoporosis, and general susceptibility to disease. For this reason, whatever the complaints of the patient, the digestive function should be given careful attention in diagnosis and treatment. If significantly impaired, it must be strengthened first before other aspects of the patient's condition can be treated.

---

[14] *In principle, all abnormalities of fluids can be considered in the context of fluid imbalance. But depending on the rest of the symptom picture, it may be more meaningful to interpret abnormalities in thirst, sweating, etc., as part of a subpattern or pattern of heat, asthenia, etc.*

[15] *Kampo fluid stagnation pathology is related to disease patterns of damp, phlegm-rheum, water swelling, etc., in Chinese medicine.*

[16] *Related to the disease patterns of splenic transformation failure and splenogastric vacuity (with damp encumbrance) in Chinese medicine.*

Weak digestive function is manifested by a chronic susceptibility to some or all of the following:[17]

- poor appetite or no sense of hunger
- little food intake (sensation that the stomach fills up quickly)
- no enjoyment in eating (insensitivity to taste)
- discomfort in the upper abdomen (uncomfortable sensation of fullness or heaviness, sensation of a lump, feeling of blockage, etc.)
- bloating, excessive eructation, or flatulence
- abdominal pain
- heartburn
- nausea, vomiting
- excessive or insufficient salivation
- diarrhea, or atonic constipation, or bitty stool
- lethargy after eating (esp. in the afternoon)

In addition, symptoms such as lusterless complexion, easy fatigability, shoulder stiffness, headaches, dizziness, insomnia, and nervousness are frequently correlated with weak digestive function.

References for Chapter 5

(1) Mori, Yūzai. *Chūigaku no Ketsuo (Blood Stasis in Traditional Chinese Medicine)*. Kobe Traditional Chinese Medicine Research Society (Reprint).

(2) Tani, Tadato. "Gendai Iryō to Kampōyaku (Modern Medical Care and Kampo Medicine)." Iyaku Journal Company, 1988, p.102.

(3) Ogawa, A., T. Ikeda, and M. Ikeda. *Kampō to Shinkyū no Fukushō: Kokon Fukushō Shinran (Kampo and Acumoxa Abdominal Signs: A New Look at Abdominal Signs Past and Present)*. Tokyo: Kampo No Tomo Company, 1989, pp.282-293.

(4) *Ibid.*, p. 285.

(5) *Ibid.*, pp. 290-1.

(6) *Ibid.*, pp. 292-3.

---

[17] *Note that many of these symptoms also suggest fluid stagnation involving the digestive system, which occurs easily when the digestive function is impaired. There is in effect a mutual interaction: Fluid stagnation, perhaps consequent to excessive food intake, can damage the digestive capability of the body; while poor digestion, in failing to move and assimilate ingested matter properly, can give rise to fluid stagnation.*

Chapter 6
The Four Examinations

In Kampo as in traditional Chinese medicine, routine diagnosis begins with the so-called Four Examinations: inspection, audio-olfactive examination, inquiry, and palpation. Each mode of examination brings to light particular aspects of the patient's condition. The goal is to correlate and synthesize all that may be perceived by looking, listening, smelling, and touching into a comprehensive character sketch of the patient's state of imbalance.

The presentation here is an abridged version of the Four Examinations, adapted for the purposes of this manual. While it is laid out sequentially, one procedure at a time to avoid undue confusion, all four procedures are interrelated and need not be performed in any particular order. A point of concern identified during the history may be confirmed by palpation. In turn, a palpation finding may lead you to question the patient on an issue glossed over previously.

What matters is that you have obtained all the information by the end. You should develop your own sequence of examinations, and with practice and experience, learn to tailor it to each diagnostic encounter.

I. Inspection

Beginning an examination with inspection is probably something common to all medical systems. As you greet the patient, many things can be learned at a glance, provided that you have trained yourself to see them and appreciate their significance.

The following characteristics should be noted during the examination:

- **General appearance**

    Stature, build, posture, overall nutritional status, dress

- **Appearance of face**

    Complexion, expression, eyes (appearance, quality of the glance, eye contact with examiner)

- **Appearance of skin (including hair and nails)**
  Hue, luster, nutritional state, pigmentation, lesion
- **Muscular development**
- **Vascular abnormality**
- **Edema, puffiness, perspiration**
- **Appearance of mobility**
  Gait, balance, range of motion
- **Demeanor**
- **Mental disposition**

Inspection of the tongue

In Kampo, tongue diagnosis is not as developed as in Chinese medicine. It is considered more important in acute diseases than in chronic diseases. The significance of the appearance and color of the tongue and tongue fur is not discussed in this manual, with the exception of signs pertaining to blood imbalances. Dark red or purple color in the tongue and (dilated) veins beneath the tongue, as well as in the lips, lining of the mouth, and gums are indicative of blood stasis (see p. 43, Blood Stasis). Paleness of the tongue, gums, and lips suggests blood vacuity (see p. 46, Blood Vacuity).

II. Audio-olfactive examination

Much information can be obtained through the faculties of hearing and smelling. Here we will limit ourselves to consideration of the following sounds:
- voice volume and quality
- breathing
- abdominal noises
- sounds expressive of discomfort and pain

Traditionally, a comprehensive examination may also include smelling the breath, the body odors, and the excreta.

III. Inquiry

The essence of Kampo inquiry, or history taking, is embodied in the traditional injunction given to medical students: "Listen to the patients, they are telling you their diagnosis." Whereas in modern medicine the reliance on diagnostic devices has tended to erode the importance of subjective account of illness, it remains central to Kampo diagnosis.

Inquiry in Kampo parallels history taking in modern medicine to a large extent. By way of sympathetic questioning, the examiner elicits a history of the illness. He or she should encourage a full report of all symptoms, including vague and seemingly unimportant ones, however tangential they may appear to the chief complaint. The examiner also delves into the patient's prior medical history and family medical history to learn about any perduring or recurrent maladies, the patient's susceptibilities, and response to medications. Attention is also directed to the patient's personality and emotions, lifestyle, and living and work-ing environment, as these psycho-socio-economic factors all bear on the genesis and evolution of illness.

Obviously, innumerable questions may be posed depending on the clinical circumstances. The guideline below simply identifies aspects of Kampo inquiry that may not be routinely included in modern medical examination, and that may involve interpretations or lines of questioning peculiar to Kampo. Note the prominence of information on appetite, digestion, thirst, excretion, sensitivities, and preferences. Although these simple host factors may often be irrelevant to the quest for specific disease entities, in Kampo they are considered to illuminate the nature of imbalance and the requisite therapy.

Selected routine areas of kampo inquiry

1. Cold and heat (see p. 38, Table 2, Cold and Heat: Comparison of Attributes)

Relevant questions include subjective sensations of and sensitivities to cold/heat, and the influences of cold/heat on symptoms. Preferences for warm-ing/cooling foods and drinks, cold/hot weather or places can also contribute to the discernment of cold/heat features in the symptom picture.

2. Perspiration

Ask about the occurrence of perspiration in conjunction with other symptoms, as well as the typical state of perspiration (e.g., tendency to excessive sweating).

The site may be significant (e.g., sweating only from the head), so may the time of the day (e.g., night sweating).

3. Urine

Ascertain any abnormality in micturition (frequency, sense of incomplete voiding, etc.) and urinary output relative to fluid intake.

It may be pertinent to ask about color if a sample is not taken. The color of urine can indicate cold/heat, as clear urine is associated with cold, and dark yel-low urine with heat.

4. Stool

Question patients on the frequency of bowel movement and any abnormality in the color, odor, consistency, and content of feces. If there is a problem, ask about the accompanying symptoms, the aggravating or precipitating factors (overeating, eating certain foods, exposure to cold, etc.), and the use and effect of medications.

5. Thirst and taste in the mouth

Lack of thirst or thirst with preference for warm drinks (even in summer) often implies cold, while thirst with high fluid intake or thirst with preference for cold drinks (even in winter) is usually a symptom of heat. Thirst with immediate vomiting of ingested fluid usually signifies fluid imbalance.

Some patients may have mouth dryness (defined in Kampo as having the desire to moisten the mouth, with little or no desire to drink); or conversely, excessive salivation.

Changes in the taste in the mouth also have diagnostic value. A bitter taste (corroborating heat) and lack of sensation of taste (signifying weak digestive function) are the only two such signs mentioned in this book.

6. Appetite, food intake, and digestion

Changes in appetite appear in various conditions. The main one dealt with in this book is poor appetite (lack of or reduced appetite) associated with digestive upsets, weak digestive function, stress, or chronic illness.

Dietary preferences or indulgences can point to certain imbalances. For example, overconsumption of alcohol and rich foods may contribute to the genesis of blood stasis and/or fluid imbalance, while overconsumption of cold raw foods or sweets can give rise to cold patterns (including coldness syndrome) and/or fluid imbalance.

The digestive function should be carefully assessed. Be alert to possible connections between GI symptoms and problems affecting other systems of the body.

7. Sleep

Apart from its routine inclusion in Kampo examination, inquiry about sleep disturbances is essentially the same as in modern medicine.

8. Head and body

If the patient experiences headaches, heavy-headedness, light-headedness, or dizziness, ascertain the nature, site, severity, duration, accompanying symptoms, and triggering factors.

With regard to the body, question the patient about any aches and pains, stiffness, paresthesias, or other discomfort in the trunk and limbs. Fatigue, weakness (limpness), or sensation of heaviness (general or localized, such as to the lumbar region, knees, or the limbs) can aid in pattern discernment.

See Chapter 7, Abdominal Examination, for more details on inquiry about chest and abdomen.

9. Gynecologic issues

History on menstruation, pregnancy, and childbirth should be routinely elicited from female patients regardless of the nature of complaint. The examiner should also ask about the volume, color, and consistency of vaginal discharges (what is normal for the patient and any abnormality).

The possibility of pregnancy should be considered. Certain remedies may provoke miscarriage and are usually contraindicated in pregnancy.

Some general Kampo interpretations of menstrual phenomena and vaginal discharge are as follows:

- Amenorrhea may signify cold, blood vacuity, or blood stasis; and as in modern medicine, pregnancy or menopause.
- Delayed arrival of menses, light flow, and pale menstrual blood generally signify cold or blood vacuity.
- Premature arrival of menses, together with a heavy flow and thick red menstrual blood, generally signify heat.

- Purplish menstrual discharge with clots implies blood stasis.
- Thin, profuse, clear, or white vaginal discharge is associated with cold; and thick, scant, yellowish vaginal discharge is associated with heat.

IV. Palpation

The practice of palpation as a form of diagnosis is common to many branches of Oriental medicine. A well-known example is pulse reading, which is also done to some extent in routine Kampo examination. However, the main form of palpation in Kampo is abdominal palpation, more developed and accorded far greater importance in Japan than its counterpart in traditional Chinese medicine.

As in Western abdominal examination, the hands are used to elicit information from the abdomen. Yet the emphasis differs. A Western physician carries out palpation and percussion primarily to evaluate the internal organs and to deduce the presence of lesions within the abdominal cavity. By contrast, the focus of interest for a Kampo doctor is not what is hidden beneath the abdominal wall. It is the wall itself: the overall tone and nutritional state, areas of abnormal tension, and other features defined by touch and applied pressure. Coupled with the patient's subjective response, the information so gathered not only contributes to the identification of pathology in traditional terms, but can also lead directly to the selection of suitable remedies.

Like pulse reading, Kampo abdominal palpation belongs to the world of sensory perception. It requires a certain measure of sensitivity, and expertise can only accrue from practice and experience. However, even a rudimentary grasp of the technique can augment the practitioner's diagnostic acumen.

Palpation of other body parts

In addition to the abdomen and chest, the limbs and other body surfaces are palpated chiefly to evaluate variation in surface temperature, characteristics of the skin, and muscular tension. This general palpation is not discussed independently.

Note that palpation of specific points is also performed by Kampo doctors trained in acupuncture.

Toward a clarification of the physiologic basis of Kampo abdominal palpation

That superficial structures can yield information about deeper or apparently remote structures is a widely appreciated phenomenon. It is the whole point of diagnostic palpation, and has its basis in the functional and structural interconnection of all body parts.

The diagnostic potential of the abdominal wall is recognized in modern medicine, which has noted many relationships between wall features and disease states. Well-known examples include:

- Muscle spasticity and tenderness overlie areas of peritoneal irritation.
- Zones of hypersensitivity of the wall skin sensory nerve fibers (Head's zones) appear to reflect specific areas of peritoneal irritation.
- Degenerative changes in the wall can indicate a subjacent chronic pathologic condition.

- Prominent venous patterns indicate vena cava obstruction or portal hypertension.
- Skin lesions may be produced by gastrointestinal diseases.
- A bluish discoloration of the umbilicus suggests intraperitoneal hemorrhage.

In Japan, other relationships are being clarified through Kampo clinical studies. In addition, recent research utilizing imaging techniques such as thermography, X-rays, and ultrasound have begun to correlate certain Kampo abdominal signs with measurable or visualizable physical changes. Such developments have instilled hope in those who recognize the clinical value of this diagnostic form but object to its lack of precision, that in the near future, it will be possible to translate Kampo abdominal palpation findings into quantitative data.

Like most elements of traditional medicine, Kampo abdominal palpation has yet to earn the sticker of scientific validation. In the meantime, Japanese physicians who incoporate Kampo in their practice attest to its usefulness, especially as a complement to modern analytic methods. For instance, restricted blood flow in the coronary artery frequently shows up as a prominent Kampo palpation finding in the epigastric region, making timely treatment possible to reverse the progression to myocardial infarction. Usually this notorious killer can neither be anticipated nor averted if one relies solely on the electrocardiograph (ECG). An example of blind spots that remain in modern clinical practice, it both reminds us of the inadequacy of technology, and warns against the neglect of "primitive" data that are gathered through the senses.

The following chapter focuses on Kampo abdominal examination.

Chapter 7
Abdominal Examination

Abdominal examination is the component of examination based on Kampo abdominal palpation.[1] Although it contributes to the classification of pathology on a theoretical level, it is first and foremost a practical, treatment-oriented diagnostic method.

The two main objectives of abdominal examination are:

1. Determination of the constitutional state, which in turn indicates the general treatment approach.

2. Where possible, the determination of suitable remedies.

Many formula patterns include particular abdominal signs. The findings of abdominal examination can therefore contribute to differential diagnosis, indicate the pertinence of a particular group of formulas, or corroborate other indications for a specific formula.

Some practitioners go so far as to consider abdominal examination the essential basis for treatment. A moderate and more judicious standpoint is to regard it as one aspect of pattern identification. Depending on the overall picture, signs gleaned with this form of diagnosis may or may not have a central significance.

I. Preliminary considerations

We have aimed to provide an introduction to Kampo abdominal examination for those unfamiliar with Oriental medicine, one that gives a sense of its scope of utility as well as its place within the practice of Kampo. To lend perspective to our presentation, a few observations are in order.

The study of abdominal examination is plagued by the ambiguity inherent in the communication of subjective observations, and by the lack of a definite methodology. Authorities differ in the interpretation of the classics, so that a sign referred to by the same name may be characterized and codified several ways.

---

[1] *In practice, the chest wall is assessed at the same as the abdominal wall, and the term designates the entire process.*

In recognition of these problems, one leading proponent of abdominal examination has developed a more rigorous method of documentation whereby, to achieve greater accuracy in the portrayal of palpation findings, pre-defined marks are drawn directly on the abdomen of the patient. A photograph is taken of the drawing, and findings so recorded at each visit can be compared and analyzed.[2]

This method is a considerable refinement over the conventional diagrammatic representations. Changes that occur in the course of treatment can be recorded with greater accuracy, new signs can be more readily distinguished from old, and principal signs from accessory ones. Over time, it becomes possible to trace the stages of evolution or devolution of a sign, and learn the therapeutic range of a remedy in terms of abdominal signs.

Improved documentation may well promote both personal mastery of abdominal examination and new advances in this age-old practice. Yet, for reasons of feasibility, the prevailing means of representing abdominal signs continues to be a combination of illustration and verbal description. This manual follows suit, for despite the limitations of the conventional method, it lends itself to an introductory treatment of the subject.

II. Terminology

The vocabulary used to locate Kampo abdominal signs is drawn as much as possible from modern medical terminology. It includes a list of anatomic structures that serve as useful landmarks (Figure 1)
- xiphoid process of sternum
- costal margin
- rectus abdominis muscle (or rectus muscle)
- linea alba (midline)
- umbilicus
- inguinal ligament (Poupart's ligament)
- superior margin of os pubis

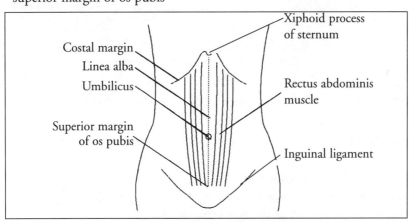

Figure 1: Landmarks of the abdomen

[2] Ogawa, A., T. Ikeda, and M. Ikeda. Kampō to Shinkyū no Fukushō: Kokon Fukushō Shinran (Kampo and Acumoxa Abdominal Signs: A New Look at Abdominal Signs Past and Present). Tokyo: Kampo no Tomo Company, 1989.

In Western abdominal examination, the abdomen is commonly divided into four quadrants (Figure 2) or nine regions (Figure 3).

References are made to these subdivisions as needed.

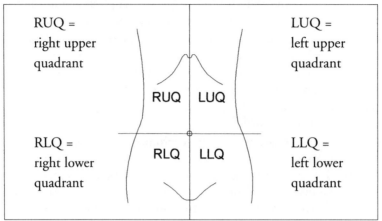

Figure 2: The quadrants of the abdomen

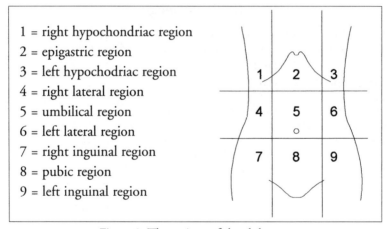

Figure 3: The regions of the abdomen

Finally, three additional designations of region are useful because a different mapping method is traditionally employed in Kampo palpation:

• **Substernal region (Figure 4)**

Comparable to the epigastric region, but extending farther down to about an inch above the umbilicus.[3]

• **Subcostal region (Figure 5)**

A zone beneath the costal margin. Includes the right and left hypochondriac regions and a portion of the epigastric region.

• **Periumbilical region (Figure 6)**

Refers to the area circumscribing the umbilicus about two finger breadths in radius.

---

[3] *More precisely, down to the acupuncture point CV-9.*

Note that, unlike modern partitions with well-defined perpendicular lines, the Kampo regions have no clear-cut boundaries.

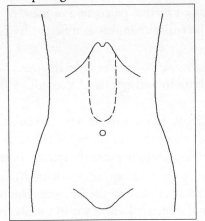

Figure 4: Substernal region   Figure 5: Subcostal region

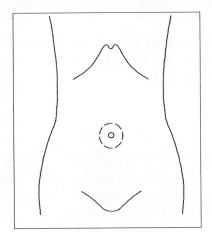

Figure 6: Periumbilical region

III. Abdominal Signs

Abdominal signs refer to significant features of the abdominal wall identified and interpreted in Kampo abdominal examination. The presentation below is restricted to signs most relevant to our consideration of climacteric disorders, and includes most of the abdominal signs emphasized in contemporary Kampo.

A. Signs more general in nature

1. Abdominal strength

The abdominal wall reflects the general fitness and nutritional status of the body. Abdominal strength correlates with many other physical indicators of reserve and resistance. For this reason, it would most likely take precedence if any one characteristic had to be relied upon to evaluate the constitutional state.

The three components of abdominal strength are the thickness of the wall, muscle tone (springiness or elasticity of the abdominal muscles), and the amount of subcutaneous fat. It is evaluated from a composite perception of these physical characteristics through palpation of the entire abdomen at different levels of pressure.

Characteristics such as thickness, resilience, good muscular development, and a fair deposit of subcutaneous fat contribute to a diagnosis of strength. A firm abdomen is an indication of sthenia.

Conversely, characteristics such as thinness, softness, poor muscular development, scant fat deposit, or obese flabbiness denote the lack of abdominal strength. A weak abdomen indicates asthenia, and may signal prolapse of the internal organs.

It is necessary to distinguish strength from guarding or spasticity. Marked tone or unusual contraction of the rectus muscles can give the false impression of firmness and sthenia. To check if the tension is merely local or superfical, also palpate inward and downward from the lateral border of the rectus muscle. If the condition is actually one of asthenia, the strength assessed this way will be appreciably less.

Consistent with the rating scale for constitutional state (p. 36), an analogous five-level scale is adopted in this manual to represent abdominal strength:

    5 = firm to very firm
    4 = moderately firm
    3 = medium
    2 = moderately soft
    1 = soft and weak

"Medium" denotes an abdomen of average strength, one that seems neither firm nor soft. Note that a woman's abdomen is in general softer than a man's. In order to develop a sense both for what "medium" is and the range of strength, it is advisable to palpate anyone willing to lend his or her abdomen for the purpose.

It may be that soft and firm are the only two levels that can be judged with confidence in the beginning. Since chronic problems are the focus here, it is prudent to make a conservative estimate when in doubt. For example, choose medium if you cannot distinguish between medium and moderately firm. More accurate determination of strength will come naturally with experience.

If only abdominal strength is used to evaluate the constitutional state, a five would correspond directly to sthenia, one to asthenia and so forth. However, reliance on any one indicator is poor practice in pattern identification. Despite its importance in constitutional state diagnosis, conclusions from abdominal strength should be tempered by other attributes of vitality.

2. Surface characteristics

The abdomen is a good place to evaluate the skin, as it presents to view a large expanse of this sensitive tissue.

Skin characteristics of the abdomen have the same diagnostic significance as the rest of the body surface, providing information about the constitutional state, the severity of illness, and the nature of pathology.

Inspect for color/pigmentation (localized discoloration, generalized color changes), luster, and nutritional status. Check the texture and the degree of moisture. Moist skin and edema bespeak a problem in fluid balance and can help you differentiate between two otherwise similar abdominal patterns. Dry or poorly nourished skin in the lower abdomen as elsewhere in the body generally signifies blood stasis or blood vacuity.

Look for evidence of subcutaneous bleeding and vascular changes such as venous dilatation and spider nevi. Scars indicating previous surgery or trauma should alert the examiner to the possible presence of adhesions, especially if they are located in the lower abdomen. In Kampo parlance, the above findings imply the involvement of blood stasis in the pathology.

A healthy abdomen is warm, with a very slight increase in the relative temperature (not easily detected by palpation) from the chest to the upper abdomen to the lower abdomen. Deviation from the norm provides further clue to the nature of the disorder and points to the appropriateness of certain substances. An abdomen cold to the touch, for example, often requires treatment with warming substances. Heat palpated in the chest suggests the pertinence of formulas containing particular cooling or anti-inflammatory substances.

3. Contour

The overall shape of the abdomen also contributes to the assignation of constitutional state.

A flat contour is common in well-nourished, athletic adults, i.e., average to sthenic constitutional states. The rounded or convex contour, with the maximum height of convexity at the umbilicus when the individual is recumbent, can be the result of excessive subcutaneous fat deposits or poor muscle tone. It is either sthenia or asthenia depending on the abdominal strength. A scaphoid or concave contour may be observed in thin persons of all ages. Resulting from a decrease in subcutaneous fat in the abdominal wall and a relaxed or flabby musculature, it signifies asthenia.

4. Infrasternal angle

The lateral spread of the ribs (as measured by the angle below the sternum formed by the right and left costal margins) suggests the general constitutional tendency. A wide angle tends to signal sthenia, and a narrow one asthenia, 60 degrees being about the average.

5. Linea alba

Though not commonly observed, broadness or a sunken appearance of the midline suggests asthenia.

6. Nature of pain

Pain ameliorated by pressure is associated in a general way with asthenia. Conversely, pain exacerbated or elicited by pressure tends to be associated with sthenia.[4]

7. Periumbilical pulsation

Pulsation is sometimes detected by laying the palm or fingers lightly on the wall in the periumbilical region. This is most often found superior to the umbilicus (or somewhat to the left), and less frequently at the position of the umbilicus or inferior to it. Figure 7 shows sample locations. It may sometimes be felt subjectively, and is occasionally a purely subjective sensation.

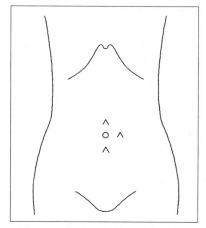

Figure 7: Periumbilical pulsations

Periumbilical pulsation appears to be closely associated with asthenia or decline in vitality, fluid stagnation, or psychoneurotic conditions. Formulas containing substances such as oyster shell, dragon bone, or poria are generally appropriate when this sign figures in the symptom picture. Examples are:

- Cinnamon Twig Decoction Plus Dragon Bone and Oyster Shell
- Bupleurum, Cinnamon Twig and Dried Ginger Decoction
- Poria, Cinnamon Twig, Ovate Atractylodes and Licorice Decoction

Sthenically-oriented formulas with pronounced diaphoretic, purgative, or emetic properties are generally unsuitable. This rule of thumb also applies when pulsation is evident anywhere along the course of the abdominal aorta.

10. Subcutaneous edema

Slight resistance in the subcutaneous layer found on light palpation of the abdominal wall (see light palpation, p. 71) most often occurs in the substernal region. It may also be noted in the subcostal region, around the umbilicus, and elsewhere in the lower abdomen.

---

[4] *The correspondence would be exact if one speaks in terms of vacuity-type pathology and repletion-type pathology as in Chinese medicine. The former is correlated with pain relieved by pressure, the latter with pain worsened by pressure.*

This phenomenon is rarely discussed in the Kampo literature despite its clinical commonness. A forerunner of resistance that involves the underlying muscular tissue, it appears to arise from disturbances in the exchange and flow of fluid within the subcutaneous tissue.

Subcutaneous edema often accompanies signs characterized by muscular resistance, and it may be all that can be detected in the early stage of such signs.

B. Signs associated with specific regions

1. Substernal region

• Substernal hard glomus

Resistance (impression of hardness or tightness) and tenderness (pain elicited by pressure) in the substernal region, together with subjective discomfort in the region – sensation of a lump (glomus) or an uncomfortable sense of fullness, oppression, etc. Local skin temperature may be palpably cooler in an asthenic patient.

This is the most common of the substernal signs. It should be checked on an empty stomach, since in healthy people a transient phenomenon resembling substernal hard glomus may occur following food intake. It is seen in both sthenic and asthenic states.

The location and extent of this sign is variable. It may be directly inferior to the xiphoid process, or more or less centered in the middle of the upper abdomen. Possibly, in patients with gastric prolapse, it is detected at the level of the umbilicus. It may first appear in the upper part of the region, enlarge, and extend downward to the lower part as a disorder progresses; or vice versa. See Figure 8 for examples.

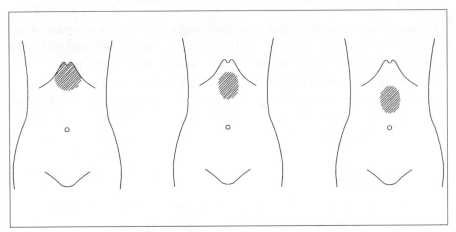

Figure 8: Substernal hard glomus

Substernal hard glomus is chiefly observed in gastric disorders, heart diseases, and other pathologic conditions of organs and tissues near the diaphragm. Depending on the pattern of symptoms and signs, formulas containing substances such as ginseng, poria, atractylodes, or bupleurum may be indicated.

Examples appearing in this book include:
- Pinellia Heart-Draining Decoction
- True Warrior Decoction
- Cinnamon Twig and Ginseng Decoction
- Major Bupleurum Decoction and other formulas containing bupleurum
- **Substernal splashing sound**

Refers to the sound of fluid moving about when the upper abdominal wall is percussed with the finger tips (figure 9). It is usually elicited in a soft abdomen, typically in the lower half of the upper abdomen.[5] Patients manifesting this sign often report an uncomfortable sense of fullness, bloating, or other feeling of discomfort in the substernal region.

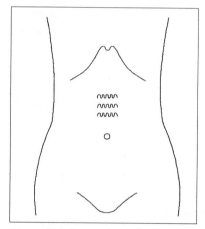

Figure 9: Substernal splashing sound

Research has associated substernal splashing sound with low tonus of the abdominal wall, position of the stomach, and presence of gas and fluid within the gastric cavity.[6] It is common in patients with gastric atony or prolapse.

Check for this sign several hours following meal intake, when food would normally have been emptied from the stomach. It can be a temporary phenomenon, but is often chronic in many fluid imbalance conditions characterized by impaired digestion, nausea or vomiting, dizziness, and headaches. Treatment of patterns featuring this sign typically calls for formulas incorporating substances such as ginseng, pinellia, poria, atractylodes, and ginger. Examples appearing in this manual include:
- Poria, Cinnamon Twig, Ovate Atractylodes and Licorice Decoction
- Pinellia, Ovate Atractylodes and Gastrodia Decoction

---

[5] May also be detected around the umbilicus.

[6] Tosa, Hiroyori et al. "A Study of the Mechanism of "Inai-Teisui" (Water-imbalance syndrome in Kampo medicine) – The First Report (Japanese), Japanese Journal of Oriental Medicine 33(2):53, 1982.

2. Subcostal region

• Subcostal distress

Resistance and tenderness beneath the costal margin. Furthermore, the fingers (the middle three are employed) of the examiner encounter resistance when an attempt is made to push them upward from under the edge of the costal margin into the thoracic cavity. This maneuver induces discomfort or pain accompanied by a suffocating sensation in the chest. In marked cases, simply pressing the subcostal area would elicit tenderness as well as discomfort or pain of a smothering nature. This sign is usually most evident around the point where an imaginary line from the umbilicus to the nipple intersects the costal arch. Additionally, cutaneous hypersensitivity (evaluated by gentle lifting of a fold of skin) and edematous tendency is often found parallel and superior to the costal margin.[7]

Subjectively, the patient may have a feeling of oppression or distressing fullness around the costal arch, or may find it oppressive to wear tight clothing.[8] Such subjective symptoms tend to be vague or absent except in high-grade manifestations of this sign.

Subcostal distress may be unilateral or bilateral, and the right side is more affected than the left in a majority of cases. The degree of manifestation depends on the nature of the disorder and the constitutional state, being more obvious in acute disorders and sthenic patients, and barely detectable in some chronic disorders or asthenic patients. Figures 10a,b,c depict three possible cases.

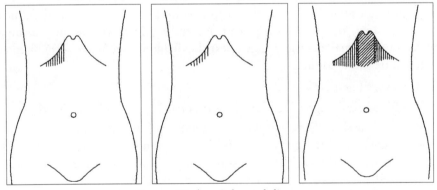

Figures 10a,b,c: Subcostal distress

10a: Medium grade, right side   10b: Low grade, right side   10c: High grade, bilateral, with substernal hard glomus

The link between this sign and liver abnormality is particularly strong, but it appears commonly in a wide variety of disorders involving the respiratory tract and structures adjacent to the diaphragm, such as the heart, stomach, and spleen. In addition, it may be an important element of the symptom picture in allergies, neuroses, gynecologic problems, and kidney disorders. Formulas with a pattern

---

7 *Hosono, Shirō. "Kyōkyōkuman o Kataru" (On the "Kyokyokuman"). (I, II, & III). Journal of Japan Society for Oriental Medicine 16:2-4, 1966.*

8 *Termed "bitter fullness in the chest and lateral costal region" in Chinese medicine.*

that includes subcostal distress therefore have far-ranging applicability. As a rule these formulas contain bupleurum. Examples in this manual are:

- Major Bupleurum Decoction
- Bupleurum Decoction Plus Dragon Bone and Oyster Shell
- Counterflow Cold Powder
- Bupleurum and Cinnamon Twig Decoction

In contemporary Kampo, there is a tendency to emphasize subcostal distress in patient evaluation, and critics of the practice decry the parallel tendency to employ bupleurum liberally. It is decidedly poor practice to prescribe a bupleurum formula whenever subcostal distress is diagnosed. One detail by itself is not enough to clinch the diagnostic conclusion. The entire symptom picture must be taken into consideration. Subcostal distress may not have therapeutic exigence. For instance, it may be an enduring vestige of a previous case of pleurisy that resulted in marked callosity of the pleura.

The subcostal region overlaps with the substernal. Subcostal distress is often accompanied by substernal hard glomus (as shown in Fig.10c), while more extreme manifestations of substernal hard glomus can "spill" into the subcostal region. Thus it may be difficult to distinguish one sign from the other, or to decide which sign has greater diagnostic significance.

One further note of caution: resistance in the subcostal region should not be automatically treated as subcostal distress, the most common sign in the chest and subcostal region. Some ten other palpation findings in the region are defined in Kampo. Liver or spleen enlargement, impending liver cirrhosis, liver or lung cancer, or other malignancies located near the diaphram should be recognized as such and treated accordingly.

3. Lower abdomen

- **Blood stasis signs** (see also the next entry, LLQ Hypersensivicity)

Resistance and tenderness in the lower abdomen (excluding the periumbilical region) is considered to signify blood stasis. One or more loci may be identified. The tenderness or pain elicited by pressure on a locus of muscular resistance often radiates and may travel upward or downward. In an asthenic patient, the skin may also be palpably cooler at the reactive locus. Subjective symptoms can include a feeling of fullness or pain.

Blood stasis signs can be located anywhere in the lower abdomen, including the area along the inguinal ligaments, the superior margin of the os pubis, and the lateral regions. But they are most commonly identified beneath the umbilicus just beyond the periumbilical region, over the sigmoid colon, and over the cecum. These sites are shown together in Figure 11. Figure 12 depicts a possible actual finding, where a U-shaped reactive zone surrounds the umbilicus.

The extent of resistance and tenderness may vary among multiple sites. Those lying deeper in the muscular layer and extending over a greater area tend to be associated with more chronic pathological changes.

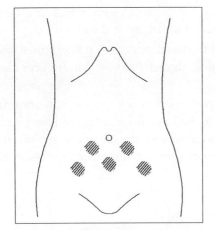

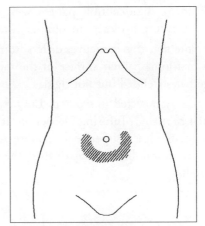

Figure 11:
Common sites of blood stasis signs

Figure 12:
Example of abdominal blood stasis findings

Abdominal blood stasis signs often precede the manifestation of distinct disease entities in the abdominal cavity, and may be the sole indication of a developing abnormality. Their identification can lead therefore to timely treatment at the pre-disease stage (refer to p. 43 for modern interpretations of and disorders associated with blood stasis).

Note that acute disorders such as appendicitis, marked nervousness, or aversion to palpation can produce similar signs, so they should not be attributed automatically to blood stasis.

Blood stasis conditions are treated with formulas incorporating substances known traditionally as:

- blood-quickening (e.g., tangkuei, moutan, ligusticum/cnidium)
- blood-cooling (e.g., rhubarb)
- blood-nourishing (e.g., cooked rehmannia, tangkuei, peony)
- stasis-transforming (e.g., peach kernel)
- antihemorrhagic (e.g., artemisia, gelatinum)
- potent "blood-breakers" (e.g., leech) for the most entrenched and recalcitrant cases.

Examples include:

- Peach Kernel Qi-Infusing Decoction
- Cinnamon Twig and Poria Pills
- Freeing Abduction Powder

• Left Lower Quadrant (LLQ) hypersensitivity

A superficial response elicited approximately in the middle of the left lower quadrant over the sigmoid colon (Figure 13).

To evaluate hypersensitivity, start near the umbilicus and move your hand swiftly and diagonally downward across the site, rubbing the surface lightly as you do so. A susceptible patient will perceive an acute pain, which can be so intense as to provoke an involuntary outcry and flexing of the knees.

Note that this maneuver differs from the usual palpation. It is executed with the first-joint palmar surface of the middle three fingers, which are kept close together, extended but not rigid.

Mostly detected in women, LLQ hypersensitivity is a specific indication for Peach Kernel Qi-Infusing Decoction. It is also regarded as a sign of blood stasis, but because it is a superficial response associated with the use of one remedy, it is by convention discussed apart from the more common resistance-type blood stasis signs.

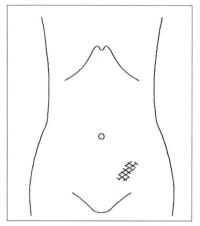 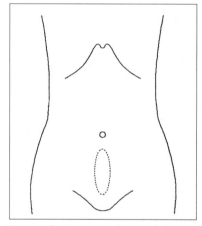

Figure 13: LLQ hypersensitivity   Figure 14: Hypotonic lower abdomen

• Hypotonic lower abdomen

Relative softness below the umbilicus (Figure 14). This hypotonicity is relative to the upper abdominal wall and the lower segments of the rectus muscles, which either manifest tension or a notably better muscle tone.

In advanced cases, a narrow depression may be visible, and palpation at an angle perpendicular to the site may reveal a conspicuous lack of normal resistance, permitting the fingers to sink easily into the abdomen. A diminished sensitivity (the lower abdomen being less responsive to touch compared to the upper) is sometimes noted by the patient and examiner alike. Local skin temperature may also be lower.

Hypotonic lower abdomen is commonly associated with functional decline and degeneration. Treatment with Eight-Ingredient Rehmannia Pills or similar formulas may be appropriate.

5. Rectus abdominus muscles

The abdominal muscles contract in response to various pathological conditions or nervous tension. This response is particularly noticeable in the rectus muscles.

Three states of rectus tension may be distinguished according to the location and extent of the muscular resistance. The significance in each case depends upon the coexisting symptoms.

- **General rectus tension[9]**

Tenseness affecting almost the entire length of the rectus muscles, extending bilaterally from the costal margin to a point somewhere between the umbilicus and the pubis (often to the lowest tendinous intersection) (Figure 15).

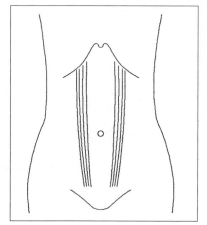 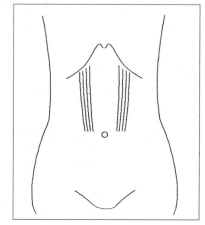

Figure 15: General rectus tension   Figure 16: Upper rectus tension

General rectus tension is commonly seen in cases of intra-abdominal pain, spasm, or inflammation, and may occur following exhaustion or psychological stress. Asthenic individuals are more likely to be affected.

Formulas containing peony are usually employed. Examples are Peony and Licorice Decoction and Counterflow Cold Powder.

- **Upper rectus tension**

Tenseness limited to the upper portion of the muscles, extending from the costal margin to about the middle of the upper abdomen or further down to the level of the umbilicus (Figure 16). Tension may reside primarily in the right or left rectus muscle, while the other member is unaffected or only slightly tense.

This form is often seen in GI disorders or conditions characterized by nervous tension. Depending on the associated symptoms and signs, formulas such as Counterflow Cold Powder, Bupleurum and Cinnamon Twig Decoction, Liver-Repressing Powder, or Pinellia Heart-Draining Decoction may be appropriate.

- **Lower rectus tension**

Tension in the lower segments of the muscles, i.e., between the level of the umbilicus and the superior margin of the pubis (Figure 17a).

---

[9] *This discussion excludes the acute abdomen or boardlike-rigidity of the abdominal wall, commonly caused by disorders requiring prompt medical or surgical care.*

Like hypotonic lower abdomen, this sign suggests a decline of sexual, urinary, or other bodily functions. Treatment with Eight-Ingredient Rehmannia Pills or similar formulas may be appropriate, particularly if it coexists with hypotonic lower abdomen (Figure 17b).

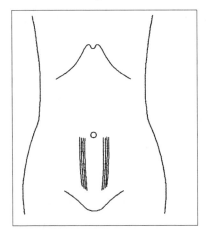

Figure 17a: Lower rectus tension

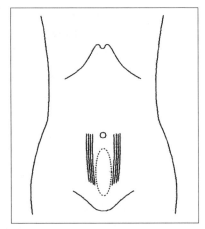

Figure 17b: Lower rectus tension and hypotonic lower abdomen

IV. Procedure

A. Preparation

Health care practitioners whose customary examination procedure requires that the patient be recumbent will find it easy to incorporate Kampo abdominal examination into their diagnostic routine. For others, the only equipment necessary is an examining table or some other similar firm surface and a good source of light.

In order to perform a satisfactory examination, the patient's abdominal musculature should be as relaxed as possible. Have the patient empty his or her bladder beforehand. The hands of the examiner should be warm. The room should be warm enough so that the patient does not shiver and tense up.

B. Position

The optimum position for the patient is supine with the legs outstretched and the arms loosely and naturally at the sides. The abdomen should be exposed from the sternum to the superior margin of the pubis. The examiner stands or sits at the patient's side (usually at the right) facing the head.

C. Inspection

Observe the appearance of the entire abdomen. Note the breadth and thickness, contour, spread of the rib cage, and surface characteristics such as skin color, nutrition, and lesions. This visual scrutiny naturally extends throughout the remainder of examination.

It is also important to look at the patient's face during palpation, not only to provide reassurance by way of sympathetic eye contact. Changes in expression such as a wince or a grimace help in the identification of reactive areas on the abdomen. Breathing rhythm may also be altered or interrupted when a sudden pain is experienced. Diagnostic value aside, such nonverbal responses alert the examiner to refrain from applying more pressure to a tender area.

D. Surface touching

Beginning at the chest and working downward, move your hand lightly over the entire abdominal wall, keeping it on the surface in a sliding motion. Avoid any quick, unexpected movement that can induce muscle tension. Note the contour, temperature, overall and local muscle tone, skin texture and moisture. Also feel for pulsations. Once you become adept, much can be learned about the abdominal strength and the foci of resistance or hypotonicity just by doing surface touching.

E. Light, moderate, and deep palpation

Note that these terms *do not* have the same meaning as in biomedical abdominal palpation.

To further evaluate the condition of the musculature and test for significant signs, palpation with the application of pressure is carried out next. Press with the end-joint palmar surface of the middle three fingers, which should be approximated, extended but not stiff. A relaxed approach is essential. Avoid quick, short jabs and any sudden movement.

Light palpation chiefly provides information at the level of subcutaneous tissue. It is performed with the fingers depressing the surface lightly at an angle 15-30 degrees to the wall. Move as if sliding from place to place, feeling for superficial resistance with the sensitive pads of your fingers. Resistance at this level is caused by abnormal accumulation of fluid in the subcutaneous tissues (see subcutaneous edema, p. 62).

Moderate palpation is done to assess the fascia and aponeuroses beneath the subcutaneous tissues and the anterior muscle layer. It is performed with the fingers at an angle 45-60 degrees to the wall. Use a gentle rolling motion in the case of thin patients. More force and a steeper angle are required in patients with substantial fat deposits. Muscular tension (felt in the fingers as a sense of resistance or hardness), laxness, and tenderness can be detected at this level.

Deep palpation is carried out with the fingers nearly perpendicular to the wall and greater pressure, in order to probe the deeper muscular structure. Areas of deeper-lying resistance and tenderness in the lower quadrants are defined with this maneuver. Marked hypotonicity will also be evident.

Although internal organs or masses may be felt and are perceived in terms of resistance and tenderness of the abdominal wall, Kampo deep palpation is not specifically concerned with their evaluation. Therefore, one neither uses as much pressure nor probes as deep as in biomedical deep palpation to assess the organs. Tenderness elicited by conventional deep palpation is often normal and should not be confused with Kampo abdominal blood stasis signs.

F. Percussion

To detect substernal splashing sound, percuss (tap) lightly with the finger tips perpendicular to the wall over the lower half of the upper abdomen and around the umbilicus. Alternatively, with the fingers touching the wall, press then release quickly several times.

G. Order of examination

Palpation of the abdomen need not follow any particular order. However, to avoid oversight and to facilitate organization of the findings, a systematic approach is desirable; for example, from top to bottom, left to right or in a spiral fashion. A possible approach is delineated below (Figure 18). (The numbers correspond to the steps in the text.)

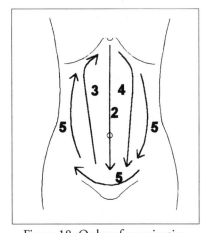

Figure 18: Order of examination

(1) Perform overall surface touching of the chest and abdomen.

(2) Moving downward along the midline, check in turn the substernal region, the area around the umbilicus, and the pubic region.

(3) Proceed from the RLQ to the RUQ along the rectus muscle. Test for subcostal distress.

(4) Repeat for the left side but in reverse order, moving from the LUQ down to the LLQ.

(5) Palpate the area along the inguinal ligaments and the superior margin of the os pubis. Conclude with the lateral regions of the abdomen.

In each area, do light palpation followed by moderate palpation. In the lower quadrants, probe deeper if muscular resistance and tenderness are not revealed with moderate palpation.

Test for LLQ hypersensitivity last, since the pain induced in susceptible persons can result in tensing of the musculature, making subsequent examination difficult.

Ask the patient to report significant reactions evoked during the examination.

H. Notes on technique

In order to have a relaxed and cooperative patient, it is important for the examiner to create an atmosphere of reassurance. Be gentle and soothing in your manner. Explanation of the examination before you start and verbal support during the examination can help to ease tension. Asking the patient to breathe slowly through the mouth can also help to promote relaxation of the musculature.

Relax your fingers. This will make them more sensitive. Do not move up and down excessively.

Although not a prescribed practice in Kampo, you may wish palpate last the sites which the patient pointed out as painful or in which you expect the greatest tenderness. This has the advantage of not causing pain and guarding (tensing of the musculature) early in the examination, and allows you to palpate the rest of the abdomen while the patient is relaxed.

Do not apply unnecessary pressure. If the area seems to be tender, approach with caution. Causing the patient excessive discomfort not only induces tension in the abdominal muscles, but also impairs rapport with the patient.

V. Summary

Below is a summary of noteworthy abdominal features introduced in this chapter:

- **Inspection**
    skin characteristics (color, luster, lesion)
    contour
    infrasternal angle
    linea alba

- **Surface touching**
    skin characteristics (moisture, texture)
    temperature
    contour
    abdominal strength
    foci of resistance
    pulsation

- **Palpation with pressure**
    Overall
        abdominal strength
        subcutaneous edema
        general rectus tension
    Chest and upper abdomen
        substernal hard glomus
        substernal splashing sound
        subcostal distress
        upper rectus tension
    Lower abdomen
        blood stasis signs
        LLQ hypersensitivity
        hypotonic lower abdomen
        lower rectus tension

VI. Medical assessment of the abdomen

To gain a more comprehensive understanding of the symptom picture, modern procedures for the examination of the abdomen may be incorporated. Inspection with reference to modern knowledge of pathophysiology naturally complements Kampo inspection. Auscultation may precede Kampo palpation. Percussion and more vigorous maneuvers to assess the organs and to identify lesions or masses deep in the abdominal cavity may be performed afterwards.

VII. Postscript

The limitation of words in teaching a skill is plain. However, the foregoing outline of signs and method should give the novice an informed start. As is true with other diagnostic skills, discriminating use of Kampo abdominal examination cannot be learned overnight. Even veteran Kampo physicians sometimes overlook signs or misinterpret findings. To cultivate mastery, the practitioner needs to conduct careful studies, meticulously correlating observation with therapeutic outcome. It is a lengthy and painstaking process. The reward will be a keen appreciation of how simple abdominal features can mirror the myriad states of health and disease, and how they can guide the practitioner to tailor treatment to individual needs.

Chapter 8
Pattern Identification

Information derived from the Four Examinations are integrated with the aid of traditional concepts of pathology to arrive at a diagnosis. This process, termed pattern identification in Kampo, is fundamentally no different from the process of disease diagnosis in biomedicine. In both cases, the practitioner endeavors to discern a pattern in the patient's condition, be it a pattern of signs and symptoms that matches a predefined formula pattern, or one produced by a particular disease entity.

For seasoned practitioners, pattern identification concurs with the process of learning about the patient. Initial contact with the patient and the medical history often suggest a list of probable patterns, which is then distilled to a final diagnosis as more information is gleaned and coalesced. This course is only possible when one has internalized a repertoire of formula patterns. For novices, pattern identification is inevitably a laborious process of comparison and elimination following the assembly of the symptom picture. It can be summed up thus:

1. Select a pattern from a pool of formula patterns, compare it with the symptom picture, and eliminate if it is not a possible diagnosis.

2. Repeat the process with the other patterns to produce the differential diagnosis – the group of patterns that could represent the patient's condition.

3. Identify the pattern that best corresponds to the symptom picture.

What qualifies a pattern to be a possible diagnosis? For a specific disease to be a possible cause of the patient's problem, some minimum combination of characteristic signs and symptoms must be present. Likewise, for a pattern to be a possible representation of the patient's condition or a facet of it, it must satisfy some threshold conditions. These are are defined as follows in this manual:

(1) Inclusion of the patient's constitutional state within the range indicated for the pattern.

(2) Presence of at least one of the major features, preferably including major abominal sign(s) (if indicated for the pattern).

(3) Presence of at least one of the minor features.

The consideration underlying the above set of criteria is to strike a balance between low risk of adverse effects on the one hand, and the flexible, maximal application of the formulas on the other. They can be relegated to the realm of discretions as the practitioner gains insight into the application of a formula. It has already been noted that (1) is often a rule of safety; (2) and (3) are based on the typical presentation of a pattern, or how the set of imbalances treated by the formula are typically manifested. The same imbalances may have alternative manifestions that are less common but still possible – the atypical presentation of the pattern.

Pattern identification draws upon the practitioner's knowledge and experience, as well as intuition. Although a pattern sometimes emerges unmistakably, it is often difficult to narrow the range of possibilities to a final working diagnosis. The standards used in Kampo being subjective and qualitative, diagnostic outcomes necessarily depend on the practitioner's perceptiveness and the weights he or she places on different facets of the patient's symptom picture. Without the independent means of confirmation available in biomedicine, a Kampo practitioner can only judge, retrospective to the treatment, whether the diagnosis is likely to have been correct.

Complexities in pattern identification

The foregoing describes a simple case in pattern identification. Often, the constellation of a patient's signs and symptoms of a case do not fall neatly into a single pattern. Diagnosis may distinguish a principal pattern plus its ramifications, or a composite of patterns. This is analagous to the occurrence of secondary conditions or complications, or the presence of multiple diseases in a patient.

Complexities in treatment

Ideally, diagnosis yields a pattern that correspond to the patient's symptoms and signs (or a subset of it). Treatment delivered by the specified formula is then said to stand in a perfect key-and-lock relationship with the pathologic condition. However, such perfect matches are relatively uncommon, since there are limited numbers of established formulas but infinite variations of ill-health. What is usually identified in real clinical situations is a basic formula pattern. The matching of a pattern is completed in the actual treatment as needed: an established formula is adapted to a particular patient's requirement by modifying the amount of its component substances, by adding or eliminating substances, or possibly by combining another formula.

The use of extract preparations precludes most traditional means of therapeutic modulation, as is discussed in the next chapter. In more complex cases involving secondary conditions or multiple patterns, treatment is determined by the nature, severity, and inter-relationship of the sub-patterns, and may require simultaneous or sequential administration of multiple formulas according to a suitable treatment strategy. Novice practitioners generally lack the extent of knowledge and experience necessary to deal with these complexities and to fully customize the treatment. Depending on the clinical circumstance, only partial treatment may be realizable in the face of these limitations.

When treatment with the basic formula is insufficient, the most expedient course for novice practitioners is generally to complete the treatment with other resources at their disposal. Actually, the reverse – the use of Kampo to modify or complete another modality of treatment – is often what is sought by Japanese physicians to fill therapeutic voids in biomedicine. In this case, the practitioner aims at the outset to identify a pattern that matches a subset of the patient's problems, the rest being treated by modern medicine. Such pooling of therapeutic resources, rather than exclusive reliance on Kampo, is illustrative of the manner Kampo is most often applied in Japan today.

The topic of therapeutic fine-tuning will be addressed further in Chapter 10, Technical Points of Therapy.

Chapter 9
Extract Therapy

Traditionally, most Kampo medications are taken in the form of decoctions (*tō* - literally, soup), the preparation of which is a time-consuming process involving multiple steps. In recent years, commercial extract preparations in the form of powders, soluble granules, tablets, or capsules have come to dominate Kampo therapy. They are a boon in terms of convenience and practicality. Yet extracts are not simply updated versions of traditional medicine. Though more concordant with our modern preferences and lifestyles, they have shortcomings of their own. It is important to examine these shortcomings, both to be aware of the limitations of extracts and to understand how they impact therapeutic strategy and outcome.

One problem with extract preparations is inherent in the manufacture process. Extracts are commonly made by evaporating decoctions under reduced pressure. The resulting concentrate is then dried and fashioned into the desired form with the addition of excipients such as lactose or starch. Inevitable loss of volatile principles occurs during the process, with resultant attenuation of therapeutic effects.

Rather than decoctions, a number of common Kampo remedies are traditionally administered in the form of powdered herbs, or pills made with powdered herbs and a binding medium such as honey.[1] Special directions often govern their use. For example, wine may be prescribed together to aid digestion and assimilation of the remedy. Yet largely for economic reasons, most makers supply formulas originally created as powders and pills as extracts of decoctions.

This is a matter for concern for three reasons. Pharmacodynamically, decoctions are most readily absorbed and assimilated by the body, pills require the longest time to digest and therefore act most slowly and gradually, while powders are intermediate. The difference in format is not accidental but part of the therapeutic intent.

---

[1] *The name is not always a reliable indication of the original format. In spite of the designation of "powder" in their names, some such Kampo formulas are traditionally intended as decoctions.*

Secondly, medications intended as powders or pills often have a high content of volatile principles or substances that dissolve poorly in water. They are thus less suitable for the extract manufacture process. Thirdly, unlike decoctions, powders and pills are rarely formulated with herbs such as licorice and ginger, which have a protective effect on the gastrointestinal tract. When made into extracts, binding mediums that prevent gastric irritation are left out and traditional directions (which again are measures intended to aid digestion and assimilation of the medication) are disregarded. Extracts of powders and pills tend to be less efficacious than the original formats, and have probably contributed to the recent rise in minor gastrointestinal side effects associated with Kampo medicine.

Non-uniformity is perhaps the biggest problem with commercial extracts. Since 1986, extract preparations covered by the Japanese national health insurance are required to be comparable to standard decoctions approved for this purpose. Specifically, for each formula, extract content of at least two indicator chemicals must be within +/- 30% of that measured in the reference decoction. The overall quality of commercial preparations has improved as a result of this regulation. Unfortunately, each maker is permitted to create its own standards. There is thus considerable variation in quality and potency among different brands of extracts.

Partly because of the lack of uniformity, definitive conclusions cannot be drawn regarding the relative efficacy of extract preparations and traditional dosage forms. The consensus among leading clinicians is that commercial extracts are on average less effective than traditional dosage forms. As may be expected from the lack of uniformity, the reduction in potency is much more significant with some brands than with others.

Since commercial extract preparations are basically fixed-ratio products, all the pros and cons associated with fixed-ratio combination drugs apply. On the one hand, the ratio has been tested empirically to insure effectiveness; adverse interactions are either not a problem or are defined. On the other hand, there is an intrinsic inflexibility of dosage, and patient groups for which a fixed-ratio drug product is intended must be carefully delineated to ensure its proper application.

In Kampo, patient groups or responder characteristics are specified by the formula pattern. But difficulties do arise when a formula needs to be modified according to the particular needs of the patient. Traditionally, the modification may involve adding or omitting herbs, or changing the dosage of particular ingredients in the original formula. Unlike traditional decoctions, ready-made extracts are not amenable to any kind of adjustment except augmentation: extracts of single herbs or another remedy may be mixed with extract of a formula, either to increase the original dosage of particular component herbs, or to add new herbs and new actions. Strictly speaking, extracts mixed this way are not chemically equivalent to corresponding decoctions. With decoctions, all components of the augmented formula are decocted together. In the case of extracts, the addenda are prepared from separate decoctions and then mixed with the extract of the base formula. Depending on the component substances, a mixture of extracts modeled after a decoction of a formula augmented according to traditional stipulations may or may not yield the expected therapeutic benefits.

The problem of overdose may also arise when available formula extracts are combined to treat a complex condition. Originally, according to a rule governing formula combination, substance(s) that appear in more than one formula should be given in the largest single dose specified. For example, if Major Bupleurum Decoction containing 1.0g. rhubarb is combined with Peach Kernel Qi-Infusing Decoction containing 2.0g. rhubarb, only 2.0g. of rhubarb should be in the final formula. This adjustment is however not possible with ready-made extracts.

Despite these problems, fine-tuning in modern Kampo therapy often takes the form of blending commonly available formula extracts to achieve or approach the desired spectrum of effects. Several reasons are apparent behind this practice. First of all, Kampo is commonly used in the context of national health insurance, and only about 150 formula extracts and very few single extracts have been approved for coverage. Clinical demands lead to the expedient of combining available formula extracts to approximate desired formulas. Moreover, modern users of Kampo are often neither familiar with the properties of single substances nor versed in the intricacies of traditional formula adjustments. There is also a contemporary tendency to use Kampo formulas on the basis of disease diagnosis and combine them in the manner of drugs, which the extract format unintentionally has facilitated.

As is clear from the above, many issues surrounding the manufacture and use of extracts preparations remain to be resolved. Nevertheless, extracts are invaluable in modern health care. They are preferred by the majority of patients for reasons of convenience, including ease of carrying and storage; and valued by health care providers for much the same reasons. Though attenuation in efficacy is a regrettable minus, it is likely to be small if one uses quality products from conscientious makers. Indeed, since most patients cannot be expected to prepare decoctions consistently and in an optimal manner, a good commercial product may in practice compare favorably to decoctions.

Chapter 10
Technical Points of Therapy

I. Complementary use of modern drugs

Modern drugs can be used to complement Kampo treatment. Conversely, Kampo formulas can be used alongside modern drugs in a variety of situations to augment therapeutic benefits, to lessen or prevent toxicities and complications, or to enable dose reduction or even complete withdrawal from drugs. In planning such a treatment program, a basic guiding principle is to minimize the overall pharmaceutical burden to the patient while optimizing the benefits of treatment.

Since herbal constituents can influence drug effects by altering their absorption pattern, Kampo remedies and drugs should be taken at least 30-60 minutes apart. In particular, iron supplements or enzyme preparations should not be taken within 2-3 hours of a Kampo remedy, which may contain appreciable amounts of tannin. Externally applied medications (ointment, inhalants, suppositories, etc.) can be used concomitantly with Kampo remedies.

Overdose may occur when Kampo remedies contain chemicals that are additive with drugs or potentiate their actions. To date, three such instances have been noted:

- The use of potassium-depleting diuretics with remedies containing licorice.
- The use of sympathomimetic drugs with remedies containing ephedra.
- The use of modern over-the-counter laxatives with remedies containing substances having laxative effects.

If the goal is replacement of drug therapy with Kampo, reduction of drug dosage should be gradual to avoid precipitating serious rebound reactions.

II. Fine-tuning of kampo therapy

Treatment of complex cases with multiple components may need to focus on one subset of symptoms at a time and proceed by stages. Inappropriate modification of a formula to counter all symptoms at once (especially where acute problems are involved) can dilute therapeutic benefits and worsen the condition.

Fine-tuning of therapy is an art based on a good working knowledge of the traditional therapeutic principles, the materia medica, and the theories of herbal combination. Students of Kampo are advised to approach formula modification by studying and following the guidelines on formula modification recorded in traditional clinical compendiums.[1] For beginners employing extract preparations, the principal course is to use one formula extract and complete the treatment with other resources when necessary.

On the other hand, certain simple adjustments can enhance the effectiveness of Kampo extract therapy in chronic disorders with many ramifications. Provided they are practiced prudently, they can significantly increase the ability of a novice to meet clinical demands with a small repertoire of formula extracts. A number of examples of combinations, adjunctive use of additional formula extracts, and supplementation of a formula extract by single herbs are noted in Parts III & IV. Drawn from traditional as well as contemporary practice, these instances of fine-tuning are safe and beneficial when applied properly.

Certainly, the few suggested measures of therapeutic refinement cannot antici-pate all possible clinical needs. Novices who wish to try combinations (whether suggested or ad-lib) should observe the following guidelines:

1) Start with one formula for the basic pattern identified. Based on patient response, assess the need for an auxiliary formula to supply different therapeutic vector(s) or possibly to broaden an existing therapeutic vector in the basic for-mula.

2) The auxiliary formula usually contains relatively few ingredients.

3) Beware of increase in component dosages, especially if the component has a higher potential for adverse effects. Combinations of two complex formulas resulting in extensive overlap of ingredients generally make little sense, and would not occur if pattern diagnosis is properly carried out.

4) Two formulas are adequate in most cases, though sometimes three are required. Administration of four or more formulas is very rare even when the patient presents with multiple chronic diseases.

5) Be aware that combination of two formulas with opposing actions is more likely to give rise to unexpected effects.

III. Acute conditions

Since acute disorders are not the focus in this manual, we note simply that treatment of acute/severe conditions generally takes precedence over treatment of chronic/mild ones. For instance, if a respiratory tract infection occurs in a patient suffering from hot flushes, on-going treament of the latter should generally be suspended until the patient has recovered from the infection. Acute flare-ups of a chronic condition are handled similarly.

---

[1] *Certain formulas introduced in this book derive from two simpler formulas traditionally combined to achieve a more complex spectrum of effects.*

IV. Dosage

A. General considerations

In Japan, the extract preparations most often come in the form of powders or granules. Generally, a fixed amount is taken daily in two or three divided doses. Each dose should be taken with roughly 100ml. of water[2], in which it may also be dissolved or suspended to approximate the original decoction if so desired.[3] Warm or hot water is desirable when the invigoration of depressed functions is part of the therapeutic goal, such as in coldness conditions. Cool water is indicated if the patient is experiencing bleeding, nausea or vomiting, or headrushes. Bitter remedies may be better tolerated if taken with cool water. If the taste is unacceptable to the patient, the extract may be given in capsule or tablet form.[4] The addition of wine can enhance the efficacy of certain remedies (noted under relevant entries in Part IV).

Unlike drugs, most Kampo remedies are in principle taken on an empty stomach, i.e., two hours after eating to one hour before a meal.[5] Exceptions include remedies for acute conditions, which can be taken on an as-needed basis; and remedies with a higher potential for GI disturbances, which may require postprandial administration (see p. 85, "Prevention of GI disturbances").

Dose-finding studies have not been performed in the US. In the absence of this information, the standard dosage is provisionally assumed to be the same as in Japan. In general, the dosage should be adjusted according to:

1) Body weight and age

Dosages should be scaled down for children and the frail elderly.

2) Constitution

It is better to start with a smaller than average dosage in patients who are delicate, sensitive, allergy-prone or have weak digestive function. Subsequent adjustment may be made based on patient response. This cautious approach minimizes the possibility of adverse effects.

3) Severity of illness

More severe conditions may require larger or more frequent doses, if improvement is slight with the ordinary dosage and the practitioner is confident in the diagnosis, and constitutional factors have been taken into account. For beginners, it is more prudent to try other therapeutic methods in this case.

---

[2] *Warm water is generally recommended for most remedies. However, this is a matter of individual preference or convenience in practice.*

[3] *The solubility depends on excipients used in particular brands of extracts.*

[4] *A suitable remedy tends to have an agreeable smell and taste to the patient, while an unsuitable remedy tends to be poorly tolerated. This should not be regarded as a definitive indicator of the aptness of therapy, since patient response differs according to individual sensitivity, attitudes about drugs, and culturally related taste preferences.*

[5] *Postprandial administration is frequently admitted in practice, as patients often find it more convenient or easier to remember to take their medicine after meals. Many practitioners consider that the efficacy is not significantly altered in most cases. This issue has not been studied experimentally.*

4) Purpose

Remedies taken as alteratives after distressful symptoms have subsided, for the purpose of improving the constitution over long-term, may be reduced both in dosage and frequency. A formula prescribed adjunctively to a main remedy may be taken in reduced amount and frequency, or on an as-needed-basis for acute aggravation of symptoms.

In the case of a combined remedy composed of two formulas, the respective dose should be adjusted according to the patient's particular needs (e.g., 1/2:1/2, 1:1/2, 1:1).

Dosage adjustment is an art that cannot be reduced to a set of rules. The actual response of the patient cannot be predicted with certainty in advance. For instance, a sthenic patient may exhibit a vigorous response to treatment and need only a minimal dosage to get well. Since subjective response is a prime indication of therapeutic aptness, patient participation in dosage adjustment is highly desirable. Furthermore, because the margin of safety is high over a wide dosage range for most Kampo remedies, patients can often be relied upon to regulate the dosage, once they are trained in the use of a formula.

B. Rhubarb and Aconite

Rhubarb and aconite are constituents in certain formulas introduced in this book. These two simples are also commonly added to a base formula at the discretion of the practitioner. Be sure to consult Appendix A for other important information regarding their use.

1. Rhubarb

Rhubarb has antimicrobial, anti-inflammatory, antineoplastic, anti-hyperlipidemic, purgative, and other effects. Its purgative effect is commonly utilized to treat constipation in patterns characterized by heat or blood stasis, principally in patients with intermediate to sthenic constitution.

Unlike most Kampo substances, the dose of rhubarb must be carefully individualized. It is not possible to determine the appropriate amount a priori. When adding rhubarb extract to a base formula to treat constipation, start with the equivalent of 0.5g. per day, then increase the dose gradually (up to 0.5g. at a time) as needed to move the bowels, at which point the dose may need to be reduced again or stopped altogether.[6] When diarrhea occurs from the use of rhubarb remedies, it should occasion a sense of relief. It is not suitable if it causes distressful diarrhea and feelings of weakness. Preferably, the patient should be instructed in its use, so she can regulate the dose based on individual reaction.

The daily dose of rhubarb varies from 0.5 to 3.0 grams in Japanese extract preparations of rhubarb-containing formulas introduced in this book. For some formulas, the amount of rhubarb in the extract may differ from brand to brand, sometimes by as much as three-fold. Since the dose of rhubarb in a ready-made formula extract may be excessive for the patient, it is desirable to start the patient on a reduced dose then make appropriate adjustment.

---

[6] *If using powdered raw rhubarb, which has a stronger purgative action, the usual dosage is 0.3-1.0g. per day. Rhubarb taken by itself as a laxative should be limited to occasional use only.*

2. Processed aconite

Aconite may be beneficial in coldness conditions or pain exacerbated by cold. Processed aconite (the *kakōbushi* of Japan) is greatly reduced in toxicity, but it should still be used cautiously. The daily dose of processed aconite varies from 0.5-1.0g. in Japanese extract preparations of aconite-containing formulas introduced in this book. At times, it may be desirable to supplement aconite in order to heighten the warming and analgesic effects of a base formula extract. Start with 0.5g. per day of processed aconite powder. Dosage may be increased gradually by 0.5g. a week as needed, to a total of 5g. per day for general uses (counting any aconite contained in the base formula).

V. Prevention of GI disturbances

Some formulas can induce GI disturbances in susceptible individuals due to certain substances they contain. These formulas are not suitable as such for persons with weak digestive function or those who experience adverse GI effects from their use. Preferably, the composition of the formula should be modified (by reducing or deleting or substituting the possibly offensive substances) in such cases. However, since this is not possible with extract preparations, one or more of the following measures may be tried when the pattern otherwise warrants the use of the formula.

A. Postprandial administration

Often a remedy that causes gastric distress when taken on an empty stomach can be safely taken after meals, possibly with a small amount of alcohol.

B. Dosage reduction

Prescribe 1/3-1/2 of the normal dosage. If well-tolerated, the dose can be increased gradually.

C. Formula combination

Combine with a remedy that strengthens the GI function and protects against the irritating effects of the offending substances. An example is Six Gentlemen Decoction (1/2 to 1 dose). Ginseng extract can also be useful for this purpose.

Formulas most likely to require such adjustments are indicated in Part IV. If precautions are not observed at the outset and mild GI disturbances ensue, suspend administration until the ill effects have passed, then try the measures outlined above.

VI. The healing crisis

As part of the healing response, mild or acute new symptoms or aggravation of the existing condition can sometimes occur at the outset of Kampo treatment following one, two, or three doses of medication. Being transient reactions that herald the start of recovery, they are what one might call a "healing crisis" in the West.

Many such symptoms are relatively predictable – for example, sweating or worsening of existing skin conditions from the use of remedies containing diaphoretics, diarrhea from formulas containing laxatives, or increased urinary output with remedies for fluid stagnation. From the standpoint of modern medicine, these are predictable adverse effects that occur as part of a drug's pharmacologic action. In Kampo, they are not viewed simply as unpleasant side-effects or failure in targeting the action of a drug to a specific tissue. They are also seen as cleansing reactions that are a positive sign of healing.

In Kampo as well as many other traditional medicial systems, cleansing or detoxification by expelling toxins and pathogens lodged in the body is considered a necessary step to reinstitute a healthy homeostasis . Therapy to accomplish this objective heightens activities of the organs of elimination, and sometimes leads to temporary worsening – a "blooming" of a developing or hitherto latent condition. An example is the Kampo treatment for rashes, which typically clears them by way of promoting their full expression.

Cleansing reactions may be rendered more mild by reduction of dosage. Their occurrence is not necessarily an indication of excessive dosage, but if the cleansing symptoms are severe, or unduly weaken or inconvenience the patient, then the dosage should be scaled back. To prevent unnecessary worry and ensure patient cooperation, it is important to explain the significance and the possible occurrence of cleansing reactions to the patient in advance.

Apart from predictable cleansing processes, a healing crisis may take the form of unpredictable reactions. Examples are vomiting from the use of laxative remedies and temporary loss of consciousness that is not part of the given remedy's normal effect. Unpredictable reactions present far greater difficulty for the practitioner. It may be impossible to distinguish such forms of healing crisis in the initial stage from mistreatment, sensitivity reactions, or toxicity. But the latter would persist or intensify if administration is continued, while a healing crisis is transitory and does not recur. Fortunately, this type of healing crisis is exceedingly rare.

When an unexpected development is suspected of being a healing response, some authorities recommend giving 1/5-1/4 of the regular dosage for two or three days. A true healing crisis would subside and the original condition take a turn for the better. On the other hand, if symptoms persist or worsen, or recur with increased dose, the remedy is in all probability not appropriate for the patient. The safest course for beginners is to interrupt administration altogether and take appropriate measures for relief.

VII. Evaluation

A. Evaluation of therapeutic benefits

Depending on the nature of the disorder and the remedy prescribed, therapeutic benefits may manifest quickly or only after long-term administration. Proper treatment should bring about improvement within several hours to a few days for acute conditions, and two to six weeks for chronic conditions. Several months may be required for perduring cases. Nevertheless, initial follow-up for chronic cases should be scheduled one week after commencing treatment. According to many reports, adverse effects due to misuse of Kampo usually manifest within the first week.[7]

---

[7] Tei, Munetetsu. "Kampōyaku no Yakuri" (The pharmacology of Kampo medicine). In "The ABC of Kampo Therapy," Journal of the Japanese Medical Association 108:5 (supplement), 1992.

Patients taking blood stasis dispelling remedies (especially formulas containing peach kernel) may pass dark clots and experience more pain and/or more flow in the first few cycles. This is a favorable sign. Its possible occurrence should be explained to the patient. However, if menstrual bleeding remains abnormally heavy, the formula is probably not suitable.

Note that remedies having purgative/expelling/dispersing actions tend to take effect sooner than remedies that are principally supplementing or intended as constitutional alteratives. Simple remedies composed of few herbs are faster in action than complex remedies made up of many herbs.

If treatment fails to produce expected improvement or if unexpected reactions occur, the case should be reassessed and other remedies considered.

B. Revision of treatment

Kampo formulas are not prescribed for hot flushes or headaches, but "a pattern of symptoms and signs that include hot flushes," or "a pattern of symptoms and signs that include headaches." Therefore, if the patient's condition changes so that a different pattern emerges, treatment must be changed accordingly.

C. Duration of treatment

Duration of treatment depends on the nature of imbalance and the needs of the patient.

For acute disorders, treatment may generally be terminated with the disappearance of symptoms. For chronic or recurrent disorders, it may be desirable to continue the treatment after the disappearance of most symptoms in order to prevent future episodes, to limit acute flare-ups or, to bring about desirable constitutional alteration over long-term use. A reduction in dosage or change of prescription or both may be necessary. This use of Kampo for preventive, alterative, or constructive (health-building) purposes should be carefully explained to patients, since understandably most people have no wish to continue taking medications once symptoms have subsided.

VIII. Patient cooperation

Various foregoing sections have already touched upon the importance of patient involvement in decision-making during the course of treatment. A few additional remarks are offered here.

The nature of Kampo medicine should be explained, so that patients have a realistic expectation of therapeutic benefits. Patients should also be prepared psychologically for the possibility of healing-crisis reactions and adverse effects (see Chapter 11 and Appendix A), and encouraged to report any unusual development. Improperly informed, patients may become unduly alarmed and terminate treatment prematurely, or persist with an inappropriate formula and fail to obtain timely professional advice.

As in other types of pharmacotherapy, the correct use of a formula depends on patient understanding and cooperation. Review the medication regimen with the patient. Be sure she understands how and when the remedy(s) should be taken, and in what amount. If the dosage needs to be adjusted, finding the optimal dosage may require that the patient take a greater awareness of the bodily processes. Patients vary in the ability to monitor their response to the remedy taken, and to make corresponding adjustment in the dosage. They should always be encouraged to contact the practitioner for consultations.

Chapter 11
Adverse Effects

Centuries of human experience have eliminated drastic poisons from the traditional materia medica. Various measures have also evolved to minimize unwanted effects of otherwise useful substances. As a result, Kampo remedies have a high safety profile. Adverse effects are infrequent compared to modern drugs. Usually, they are mild and subside without aftermath upon discontinuation of the medication.

The list below summarizes adverse effects that have been reported in conjunction with Kampo remedies or single substances:

1. GI effects

The most common type of adverse effects associated with Kampo remedies appear to be GI effects. They include anorexia, epigastric distress, bloating, heartburn, abdominal pain, diarrhea, constipation, etc. Often they serve as early warning signs that the formula is inappropriate. Individuals with weak digestive function are more prone to such reactions. Those with lactose intolerance may develop diarrhea from the lactose used as excipients in many brands of extracts.

2. Dermatologic effects

Reactions include skin eruptions, pruritis, or exacerbation of existing skin conditions. Allergic individuals are more susceptible to such symptoms when taking formulas having a high content of essential oils.

3. Nervous system effects

These include headache, dizziness, headrushes or flushing, drowsiness, insomnia, palpitations, numbness and tingling, chilliness, unpleasant sensation of heat, sweating, etc.

4. Other effects

Edema, hypertension, pseudo-aldosteronism, increased urination, thirst, sensitivity reactions, and other idiosyncratic reactions have been noted.

In general, adverse reactions can arise in the following situations:

1. Unwise formula consumption

Uninformed self-medication or inappropriate medication-taking practices can cause adverse reactions.

2. Symptomatic application

Using a Kampo formula like a drug to treat a disease or symptom, without due consideration for the pattern of indications, can result in adverse reactions.

3. Overdose

The wide use of extract preparations have contributed to the greater incidence of adverse effects due to overdose in recent years. First of all, novice practitioners of Kampo may prescribe multiple formulas for multiple diseases without duly noting the overlap of substances, ending up with multiple dosages of a particular substance. Secondly, since very few single herb extracts are covered by the Japanese national health insurance, substitutions sometimes are made in order to qualify for reimbursement. For example, Ginseng Combination (an approved extract) may be substituted for ginseng when the addition or increase of latter is desired. Unneeded substances get included, and undesired dosage increase of certain substances may occur as a result. This is not merely an artifact of the reimbursement system in Japan. Conceivably, it can occur for reasons of expediency, i.e., substitution of a formula extract on hand for an unavailable single extract.

Dose-related adverse reactions may also arise because the patient is more sensitive to a substance or formula than the average person. The problem disappears when the standard dosage is scaled back to a suitably low dose.

4. Interactions between substances

Undesirable effects from interactions between substances may occur from injudicious modification of a traditional formula, or improper combination with other Kampo remedies or pharmaceutical drugs.

5. Diagnostic inaccuracy

Administration of an inappropriate remedy may result in worsening of the condition or appearance of new symptoms or both.

6. Slight mismatch

Traditionally, a formula is customized in the actual treatment as needed. If not, mild adverse reactions (frequently mild GI effects) can occur when the basic pattern diagnosed is slightly at odds with the symptom picture. These are not really diagnostic mistakes, but more properly a problem of formula fine-tuning. Given the extract format and the deficiency in skills of a large number of new practitioners, the necessity of modification is often unanticipated or cannot be fulfilled, and such side effects have become possible risks associated with the "reasonable" application of formula extracts.

7. Sensitivity reactions

These generally take the form of allergic rashes. Although rare, serious hyper-sensitivity reactions leading to inflammation of liver or lung have been reported.

8. Healing crisis

For further discussion on this topic, see Chapter 10, Section VI.

In conclusion, it should be emphasized that a high safety profile is not synonymous with complete freedom from potential problems. As with any other medications, Kampo remedies can give rise to undesired results, especially if used inappropriately. While the adverse effects are generally mild, the possibility that serious allergic reactions can also occur must not be forgotten. Please consult the Caution List (Appendix A) for a roster of component substances associated with adverse effects.

Chapter 12
The Road to Mastery

K ampo formulas often have some therapeutic effect even when used in the manner of drugs, i.e., given for a disease or symptom without careful deliberation of individual factors. In certain conditions, it is possible to achieve a fair success rate just by giving a formula that is statistically likely to be effective. For example, the Polyporous Decoction pattern being common in cystitis patients, indiscriminate administration of Polyporus Decoction for cystitis can effect a cure in about 50% of the cases. Although such an approach can serve the beginner, it misses the point of Kampo therapy altogether and is prone to unwanted effects.

Ideally, one should become familiar with the empirical properties and experimental pharmacology of the ingredients in a formula. A good reference text on the materia medica can be consulted (see Bibliography). Short of this, review the content of the formula, check for substances on the caution list (Appendix A) and take appropriate precautions. For example, rehmannia can cause GI disturbances in patients with weak digestive functions. Knowing this enables the practitioner to choose other formulas for such patients or take other preventive measures. Where combination is deemed necessary, know which substance is being given at a higher then usual dosage. Adverse effects are more likely when a substance on the caution list (Appendix A) is given in large doses.

The temptation is often strong in the beginning to prescribe a combination of formulas so as to "cover" all symptoms and signs. Against this impulse, serious students of Kampo should strive to identify and administer a single formula that address the overall condition (or a subset of the symptom picture), which permits a clearer appraisal of the correctness of the diagnostic interpretation and the therapeutic effects of each remedy. The therapy can be refined subsequently based on patient response. Neophytes who prematurely resort to combinations may be unable to separate the effects of one remedy from another and never acquire the knack of pattern diagnosis. Worse, inappropriate combinations may nullify the therapeutic benefits and even give rise to adverse effects.

In order to cultivate clinical acumen and build a secure base of experience, it is a good idea for a beginner to devote special attention to one or two formulas at a time. Memorize the corresponding pattern, apply the formula whenever possible, and make meticulous observations. Compare cases where patients responded well with cases that failed to improve as expected. Invaluable principles of therapy can be learned this way, and persistence in such critical analyses will reward the practitioner with a keen appreciation of the formula's scope of applications.

PART III
KAMPO TREATMENT FOR COMMON DISORDERS RELATED TO THE CLIMACTERIC

INTRODUCTION AND GENERAL CONSIDERATIONS

The climacteric is far from a fixed entity. Its manifestation varies enormously across women, resulting from the interplay between biological, psychological, and sociocultural factors. It is thus convenient to deal separately with the common facets of climacteric symptomatology:

- Hot flushes and other vasomotor manifestations
- Sleep disturbances
- Emotional distress[1]
- Headaches
- Abnormal bleeding, vaginal symptoms
- Urinary disorders
- Body aches and pains
- Osteoporosis
- Atherosclerosis (hypertension, hyperlipidemia)

For each category of problem, the principles of treatment are described, followed by guidelines for the evaluation of efficacy, duration of treatment, and conjunctive use of modern medication. Self-help measures for the patient are also included in some cases. A table to facilitate identification of suitable formulas concludes each discussion.

I. How to use the treatment guidelines

Since the constellation of symptoms may range over several categories, we recommend approaching therapeutics by the dominant complaint of the patient. Read the discussion pertaining to the problem, then select a possible remedy or remedies from the appropriate table (see below, Quick Reference Tables). Next, consult the corresponding entry(s) in Part IV to determine whether the chosen formula pattern is an adequate description of the patient's condition. (Preliminary Considerations at the beginning of Part IV provides information essential for the proper interpretation of the entries.) Iteration of this process may either turn up the most suitable remedy, or uncover the necessity for further deliberation.

---

[1] The expression "emotional distress" has been adopted here to denote mood disorders as well as mild, non-psychotic psychiatric disorders.

The Index contains both Kampo and biomedical terms and may thus be used to direct one's research of particular diseases, symptoms, and their combinations.

Since many formulas have constitutionally balancing effects, their effectiveness may extend over several categories. In fact, some have wide-ranging applicability and appear in nearly all the tables. One formula can often take care of both climacteric problems as well as pre-existing conditions. For example, for patients who fulfill the indications for Cinnamon and Atractylodes Pills, the remedy not only treats the range of climacteric symptoms from hot flushes to myalgia, but also appears to be beneficial in endometriosis, hypertension, atherosclerosis, blood-clotting abnormalities, liver disease, and migraine headaches – in short, conditions that cause physicians to hesitate in prescribing hormones.

The patient's main complaint can often guide you to the right table. If you do not find a suitable formula there, it may be that you need to size up the case differently, either by re-ordering your evaluation of patient complaints, or by probing beyond those complaints. For example, a case presenting as urinary disturbance may be a consequence of psychological problems that have eluded the first analysis.

As stated previously, a perfect match between the patient's condition and a ready-made extract preparation is relatively rare. This introductory manual only deals with some 60 formulas and touches tangentially on the additions of substances. Explicitly suitable formulas will therefore not be found for some patients. In such cases, it may be possible to initiate the healing process by treating the constitutional factors or a subset of the symptom picture.

It must be emphasized that in presenting Kampo treatment by problem categories, we are not advocating the use of a specific symptom or disorder as the determinant for therapy. As related previously, what matters is the *pattern*. The categories are merely a convenient index to the patterns and their corresponding remedies.

Shorthand notations are convenient in refering to the following two groups of remedies:

A. Blood stasis formulas

These are formulas with appreciable blood stasis dispelling effects:
- Peach Kernel Qi-Infusing Decoction
- Freeing Abduction Powder
- Cinnamon Twig and Poria Pills
- Rhubarb and Moutan Decoction
- Supplemented Free Wanderer Powder
- Tangkuei and Peony Powder
- Channel-Warming Decoction

B. Bupleurum formulas

These are formulas containing the substance bupleurum and whose pattern of indications typically includes the abdominal sign of subcostal distress:

- Major Bupleurum Decoction
- Bupleurum Decoction Plus Dragon Bone and Oyster Shell
- Counterflow Cold Powder
- Bupleurum and Cinnamon Twig Decoction
- Bupleurum, Cinnamon Twig and Dried Ginger Decoction
- Supplemented Free Wanderer Powder

II. Quick reference tables

The tables are intended as a preliminary screening tool to help you select the appropriate remedies.

The elements of the pattern appear in the order of Constitutional State, Abdominal Findings, Other Features, and Remarks. So that the potential remedies can be quickly narrowed, the list of signs and symptoms is kept to a minimum. Only those permitting the elimination of unsuitable formulas and facilitating differentiation between similar formulas are included. They are usually major features of the pattern. Some are listed in the "Remarks" area in order to reduce cluttering.

Darkened squares indicate the range of constitutional state, and circles are used to designate the other items applicable to each formula. An item is circled for a particular formula if (1) it is a sign or symptom of principal significance, or (2) it contributes to differential diagnosis. Items not circled for a particular formula are not necessarily excluded from its pattern.

Formulas most frequently used in Japan are identified by asterisks. They tend to be remedies that are safe to try when indications are unclear. This information is provided purely for reference. It may have little pertinence for US populations living in diverse climatic and geographical conditions.

Additional remedies that may be applicable are enumerated at the bottom of the table. Consult these in Part IV if none of the formulas in the main list are suitable.

III. Other considerations

A. Self-help

Women should be encouraged to take an active role in individualizing their treatment program through healthful diet changes, exercise, stress-reduction, and other techniques for the promotion of wellness. An exemplary source of information for such self-help measures is *The Menopause Self Help Book* by Susan M. Lark, M.D. (see the Bibliography).

B. Nutrition and digestion

Proper nutrition is an important component of any healing program. Improper eating habits and addiction to legal drugs (notably caffeine, tobacco, and alcohol) not only spawn and perpetuate a number of disorders but also interfere with the realization of the therapeutic benefits.

Practical guidelines on nutrition in the perimenopause can be found in Lark's book cited above. Although this manual does not furnish a comprehensive discussion of digestive therapy, many Kampo formulas introduced here have beneficial effects on digestion and bowel function.

C. Fatigue

Fatigue has not been taken up as an independent topic. Where fatigue is a common part of the symptom picture, it is included in the pattern of the individual formula. It also appears in the tables when it is a dominant symptom contributing to differential diagnosis.

Chapter 13
Hot Flushes and Other Vasomotor Manifestations

The signature complaint of menopause in the West, hot flushes occur in some 85% of perimenopausal women, 25% of whom have them severely enough to seek medical care.(1) They may begin months or even years before the final menstrual period, but the majority of women have them after the actual menopause. They generally subside after one or two years, but can continue for five years, and even beyond ten years in a small fraction of postmenopausal women.(2,3)

Hot flushes are usually described as a sudden sensation of heat in the upper body, especially over the upper chest, neck, and face, often with visible reddening of the skin. An episode may be accompanied by profuse perspiration and followed by chills. Though harmless, they can be distressing and disruptive. Other associated symptoms include palpitations, headaches, dizziness, weakness, paresthesia (sensory changes such as numbness, tingling or crawling feeling, often in the arms and hands), cold hands and feet, and nausea. Like hot flushes, they are considered to be manifestations of vasomotor instability. The underlying mechanism has yet to be clarified, but it appears to involve a sudden downward resetting of the hypothalamic thermostat.(4)

Hot flushes vary considerably in duration and frequency. An episode usually lasts from thirty seconds to five minutes, but can extend up to an hour.(4,5) Occurrence may range from no more than one to two times a week to as many as thirty to fifty times a day. They may be most severe at night, disrupting sleep and contributing to fatigue and mood disorders. They also tend to be more pronounced during hot weather and periods of tension. In susceptible women, almost any substance, condition, or activity that raises body temperature and/or causes capillary dilation can precipitate hot flushes.(5)

Kampo treatment

With its emphasis on restoration of equilibrium and subjective wellbeing, Kampo can be most beneficial for vasomotor instability. Therapy can help to smooth out the hormonal and physical changes that occur during the climacteric years, relieving not only vasomotor symptoms, but also the many nonspecific symptoms believed to stem from psychological stress and imbalances in the autonomic nervous system.

Among the Kampo remedies listed in the accompanying table, Supplemented Free Wanderer Powder is perhaps the formula most frequently prescribed for vasomotor and other symptoms affecting perimenopausal women. It is generally a safe formula to try in women of medium to somewhat asthenic constitution.

A. Evaluation of treatment

Long-term treatment on the order of several months is the rule, but signs of improvement should be seen within 2-3 weeks after administration of an appropriate formula. The patient should feel better in general, and the frequency and severity of hot flushes should decrease.

B. Combination with conventional medication

Hormone replacement therapy is faster-acting than Kampo medicine. In cases of severe hot flushes, it can be administered alone or with an appropriate Kampo remedy for swift control of symptoms, then tapered off gradually with the aid of Kampo.

Self-help measures for the patient

A. Nutrition

Desultory eating habits that cause sharp spikes in blood-sugar levels can exacerbate hot flushes. Spicy food, hot drinks, or excessive caffeine, alcohol, or sugar can affect the body's temperature control mechanism and trigger hot flushes. Ingestion of these foods should be reduced or avoided.

B. Clothing

Heat intolerance is a feature of vasomotor instability. Advise patients to dress in layers that can be removed as needed.

C. Exercise

Regular exercise can help to reduce the occurrence of hot flushes by exerting a stabilizing influence on the autonomic nervous system. Moderation is advised, since vigorous activities can precipitate acute vasomotor symptoms, especially if undertaken suddenly by someone of poor physical fitness.

HOT FLUSHES

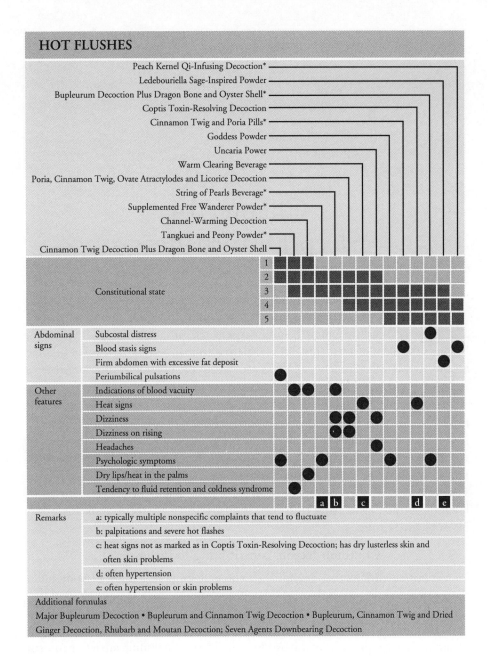

		Cinnamon Twig Decoction Plus Dragon Bone and Oyster Shell	Tangkuei and Peony Powder*	Channel-Warming Decoction	Supplemented Free Wanderer Powder*	String of Pearls Beverage*	Poria, Cinnamon Twig, Ovate Atractylodes and Licorice Decoction	Warm Clearing Beverage	Uncaria Power	Goddess Powder	Cinnamon Twig and Poria Pills*	Coptis Toxin-Resolving Decoction	Bupleurum Decoction Plus Dragon Bone and Oyster Shell*	Ledebouriella Sage-Inspired Powder	Peach Kernel Qi-Infusing Decoction*
Constitutional state	1	■	■	■											
	2	■	■	■	■	■	■	■	■						
	3		■	■	■	■	■	■	■	■	■	■	■	■	
	4						■	■	■	■	■	■	■	■	■
	5									■	■	■	■	■	■
Abdominal signs	Subcostal distress												●		
	Blood stasis signs										●				●
	Firm abdomen with excessive fat deposit													●	
	Periumbilical pulsations	●													
Other features	Indications of blood vacuity		●	●		●									
	Heat signs							●				●			
	Dizziness					●	●		●						
	Dizziness on rising					●	●								
	Headaches								●						
	Psychologic symptoms	●			●					●			●		
	Dry lips/heat in the palms			●											
	Tendency to fluid retention and coldness syndrome		●												
					a	b		c				d		e	

Remarks

a: typically multiple nonspecific complaints that tend to fluctuate

b: palpitations and severe hot flashes

c: heat signs not as marked as in Coptis Toxin-Resolving Decoction; has dry lusterless skin and often skin problems

d: often hypertension

e: often hypertension or skin problems

Additional formulas

Major Bupleurum Decoction • Bupleurum and Cinnamon Twig Decoction • Bupleurum, Cinnamon Twig and Dried Ginger Decoction, Rhubarb and Moutan Decoction; Seven Agents Downbearing Decoction

Chapter 14
Sleep Disturbances

P oor sleep is a common phenomenon in the general population, as reflected in the widespread use and misuse of hypnotic drugs. Though usually a secondary condition, it is readily perpetuated in a vicious cycle and often becomes the focus of a patient's distress. Sleep disturbances may develop or become accentuated in the perimenopause, on account of the physiological changeover as well as stressful major life events that tend to coincide with this period.

As Shakespeare put it, "sleep knits the raveled sleeve of care." Deficit in this fundamental human requirement can lead to numerous psychosomatic problems. Insomnia is second only to hot flushes as the problem that spurs perimenopausal women to seek medical help. Patients may experience difficulty in falling asleep, nightly awakenings, early morning awakenings, sensitivity to noise, inability to sleep once awake, sleep disturbed by dreams, poor quality of sleep, or any combination of these. Successful treatment begins with an appreciation of the possible etiologic factors.

Common factors contributing to insomnia

Various conditions that disrupt the neuroendocrine regulation of body functions can create sleep disturbances. The most common cause is psychological turmoil, characterized by high levels of autonomic activity. This state of increased arousal causes difficulty in initiating sleep or staying asleep. Not surprisingly, insomnia is a symptom of many psychiatric illnesses, including anxiety neurosis, depression (sufferers typically wake early in the morning), schizophrenia, and dementia.

Sleep disturbances may also be produced or aggravated by physical pain or discomfort. Migraine headaches, asthma, ulcers, arthritis, backaches, restless legs, faulty digestive function, hypertension, heart disorders, diabetes, and kidney disease are some common medical conditions in which insomnia may figure as a symptom. Nightly hot flushes are an obvious culprit in the perimenopause. They can awake the woman with heat and perspiration. Moreover, as shown by studies conducted in sleep laboratories, mini episodes of hot flushes may be subliminal, and interfere with normal rapid eye movement (REM) without causing overt sleep disruption.(8a)

Another common obstruction of restful sleep is adverse environmental stimuli, in the form of noise, light, heat, cold, humidity, an uncomfortable bed or pillow, and so forth. Elements of lifestyle and diet may also bear on the problem. Lack of exercise, poor nutrition, too much coffee or other stimulants taken in the evening, or an erratic sleep-wake schedule can all cause or exacerbate sleeplessness.

Drugs are a factor in some cases. Difficulty sleeping can result from the use of drugs such as bronchodilators, amphetamines, steroids, stimulating antidepressants, and beta blockers. Chronic use of sleeping pills often has adverse effects on the sleep pattern as well as the quality of sleep. A bout of insomnia may be part of the syndrome of withdrawal from hypnotics, tranquilizers, and antidepressants.

To formulate an effective treatment plan, the practitioner must assess all such factors that impinge on the patient's sleeping problems.

Kampo treatment

Although pharmacological experiments have documented the hypnotic, sedative, or antidepressive effects of some Kampo remedies used in insomnia, they are decidedly weak compared to those of modern medications. Rather than simple head-on sedation, which is of limited duration and benefit, Kampo medicine aims to rectify underlying imbalances. Resolution of insomnia then goes hand in hand with improvements in general health.

Insomnia during the climacteric years, with symptoms such as night sweats, waking up tired, or hot and cold spells may be largely an extension of vasomotor instability. The condition may be resolved by a formula that helps to relieve hot flushes. Some of these also appear in the accompanying table. Others can be consulted in the foregoing section on hot flushes.

Since poor sleep can be an extension of dysphoria, remedies introduced in the next chapter on emotional distress are all potentially applicable. In any case, an appropriate remedy or combination of remedies should be selected through a comprehensive evaluation of somatic and psychological symptoms.

Unlike sleeping pills, Kampo remedies are in general taken 2-3 times a day, not just before sleep. However, the dosage schedule should be adjusted to meet patient needs. In a given case, an occasional dose before retiring at night (possibly as an adjunct to a main remedy) may indeed be adequate.

Being a multidimensional problem, insomnia may require counseling, psychotherapy, or other modalities of treatment. Appropriate referrals should be given where necessary. On the other hand, coupled with reassurance to allay fear of insomnia, supportive advice, and some general self-help measures (see below), Kampo can help to initiate a turnabout in cases resistant to other therapies.

A. Issues of addiction and side effects

Used with prudence, Kampo remedies rarely cause adverse side effects. They do not produce dependence, abnormal sleep patterns, daytime sedation, malaise, or unsteadiness, neither are they associated with rebound phenomena or behavioral side effects. They can be a viable alternative for the elderly insomniacs, in whom age-related impairment of renal and liver functions increase the likelihood of retention of hypnotic drugs and resultant side effects.

B. Evaluation of treatment

Kampo remedies are not quick-acting sleeping pills. They generally bring about gradual cures over weeks or even months in recalcitrant cases, but a preliminary evaluation of efficacy is usually possible after two weeks of treatment. Even if improvement in insomnia per se is slight, the symptom picture as a whole should begin to show definite progress.

C. Combination with conventional medication

Kampo remedies may be combined with drugs if a quicker result is desired. It is possible thereby to reduce the dosage of drugs, and eventually discontinue their administration. In cases of dependency on sleeping pills, the switch-over to Kampo therapy is often difficult and should be accomplished gradually.

Drugs such as bronchodilators, amphetamines, steroids, stimulating antidepressants, and beta blockers are known to cause sleep disturbances. The use of such drugs should be reviewed.

Kampo can also be a good support measure for counseling and other modes of treatment.

Self-help measures for the patient

A. Nutrition

Strong tea, coffee, colas, cigarettes, and other stimulating substances should be avoided or minimized in the evening in patients susceptible to their effects.

Digestion can impede sleep. Avoid eating a heavy meal less than 3-4 hours before going to bed.

Patients who use alcohol to help themselves sleep should be reminded that too much alcohol is associated sleep disorders, particularly with difficulty staying asleep.

B. Exercise

Regular exercise improves overall health and promotes restful sleep. But because of its arousing effect, it should not be undertaken close to bedtime.

C. Others

Although sleep cannot be forced, it is helpful to establish a fairly regular schedule for retiring at night. Mind and muscle relaxers such as leisurely walks, long tepid baths, massages, and soft music may be incorporated into a bedtime routine according to individual inclination. Try to minimize adverse environmental stimuli such as noise, light, and uncomfortable temperature. Too hard or too soft beds and pillows should be corrected, as bad sleeping posture creates muscular tension.

SLEEP DISTURBANCES

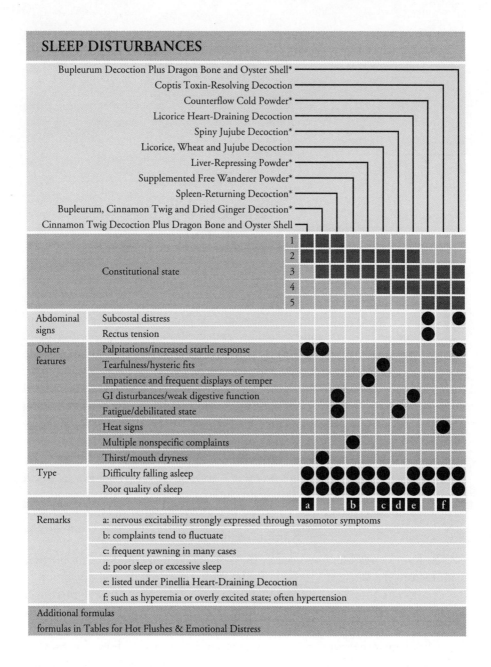

		Cinnamon Twig Decoction Plus Dragon Bone and Oyster Shell	Bupleurum, Cinnamon Twig and Dried Ginger Decoction*	Spleen-Returning Decoction*	Supplemented Free Wanderer Powder*	Liver-Repressing Powder*	Licorice, Wheat and Jujube Decoction	Spiny Jujube Decoction*	Licorice Heart-Draining Decoction	Counterflow Cold Powder*	Coptis Toxin-Resolving Decoction	Bupleurum Decoction Plus Dragon Bone and Oyster Shell*
Constitutional state	1	■	■	■								
	2	■	■	■	■	■	■	■	■			
	3		■	■	■	■	■	■	■	■	■	■
	4						■	■	■	■	■	■
	5									■	■	■
Abdominal signs	Subcostal distress									●		●
	Rectus tension									●		
Other features	Palpitations/increased startle response	●	●									●
	Tearfulness/hysteric fits						●					
	Impatience and frequent displays of temper					●						
	GI disturbances/weak digestive function			●					●			
	Fatigue/debilitated state			●				●				
	Heat signs										●	
	Multiple nonspecific complaints				●							
	Thirst/mouth dryness		●									
Type	Difficulty falling asleep	●	●	●	●	●	●		●	●	●	●
	Poor quality of sleep	●	●	●	●	●	●	●	●	●		●
		a			b		c	d	e		f	

Remarks	a: nervous excitability strongly expressed through vasomotor symptoms
	b: complaints tend to fluctuate
	c: frequent yawning in many cases
	d: poor sleep or excessive sleep
	e: listed under Pinellia Heart-Draining Decoction
	f: such as hyperemia or overly excited state; often hypertension

Additional formulas

formulas in Tables for Hot Flushes & Emotional Distress

Chapter 15
Emotional Distress

The majority of epidemiological studies show that emotional distress is not more prevalent during the climacteric.(6) Nevertheless, dysphoric symptoms such as irritability, anxiety, and depression can be prominent in women who seek medical help during the perimenopause. The complaints are usually multiple and nonspecific, and tend to fluctuate.(4) They should not be automatically considered ramifications of neuroendocrine changes and related sleep loss. Other likely causes are critical midlife problems, inadequate coping strategies, negative beliefs about menopause, and ambivalence toward aging in our youth-oriented culture.(6,7)

Emotional symptoms have an impact on the general functioning of the body and, if unresolved, can eventually promote disease processes. Disorders in which emotional distress is believed to be a contributing factor include hypertension, cardiovascular disease, chronic headaches, asthma, ulcers, allergies, and possibly cancer.

Kampo treatment

The Kampo treatment philosophy for psychological or emotional problems is distinct from the Western approach. In the West, the psychological dimension of the condition commands the focus of attention. Treatment aims at the direct improvement of emotional and cognitive dysfunctions and behavioral disturbances. In contrast, Kampo conceives of such disorders as fundamentally no different from any other type of illness: as states of imbalance with varying somatic and psychological components. Emotional symptoms are only one element in the total picture, not necessarily given more weight than somatic ones in diagnosis and treatment.

Kampo therapy in the realms of psychology and psychiatry is in principle effected through the somatic pole, by way of pharmacotherapy. The traditional theoretical justification of this approach is the mind-body unity manifested in bidirectional linkages between patterns of psychological symptoms and patterns of somatic disturbances. This concept finds modern echoes in the contemporary understanding of the interactive relationships between physiologic changes and emotional states.

Perhaps because of the somatic bias intrinsic in its therapeutic focus, Kampo treatment is generally more effective in conditions where somatic factors are significant. Many cases of emotional distress during the climacteric certainly fit this category. Another good example is depression in older people, in which psychologic symptoms are often less evident, while somatic symptoms are more emphatic. In cases where personality or environmental factors are marked, Kampo is better as an adjunct to psychotherapy.

Kampo remedies are weaker and have less defined effects than psychotropic drugs. The latter are generally preferable for alleviation of acute symptoms. Modern diagnostic labels such as depression, anxiety disorder, somatization disorder, etc., do not govern the selection of remedies, which should be based on a comprehensive evaluation of all symptoms and signs.

A. The issue of side effects

Kampo remedies have a high margin of safety. Unlike psychotropic drugs, they will not cause drowsiness, lethargy, impaired judgement, slowing of motor reflexes, or dependency. They are good options in asthenic patients or those with gastrointestinal problems, in whom drugs are more likely to cause side effects. They are particularly useful in conditions in which drugs are contraindicated, such as disorders of the heart, liver, or kidneys.

Effective dosage of psychotropic drugs can vary greatly among individuals, so that the dosage must ordinarily be adjusted by a specialist. With Kampo medications, individual difference in effective dosage is ordinarily no more than 2-3 times. They can safely be prescribed by a general practitioner for psychosomatic problems in climacteric patients and in the wider population.

B. Other approaches

There is a limit to pharmacotherapy in emotional problems. This is also true with Kampo. Counselling, psychotherapy, and support groups may be necessary to resolve underlying conflicts.

The role of stress in the etiology and severity of menopausal complaints must not be overlooked. Many menopausal symptoms can also be symptoms of stress. Flushing, for example, is a common manifestation of anxiety, and anxiety will often aggravate hot flushes during the climacteric. Relaxation and stress reduction techniques can thus be very beneficial. Even a simple expedient like exercise can help to promote emotional wellbeing and alleviate symptoms.

C. Evaluation

Improvement is generally observed within two weeks of therapy. Somatic symptoms may improve before psychologic ones. Treatment may need to be continued for two to three months, and in some cases, six to twelve months, depending on the condition.

D. Combination with conventional medication

Kampo medicine by itself may be adequate in mild cases. In more serious cases such as depression with psychotic and suicidal ideations, a comprehensive approach incorporating psychotherapy as well as drugs is imperative.

There are different possibilities of combining drugs with Kampo remedies. One can start immediately with a combination, or introduce Kampo at a later stage. Adjunctive use of Kampo may potentiate drug efficacy and reduce adverse reactions, and may enable a gradual withdrawal from drugs without rebound effects.

Kampo can also be tried specifically to alleviate untoward drug effects such as dry mouth or thirst, dysuria, menstrual disorders, tremor, dizziness, headaches, constipation, and liver disorders.(9) Formulas introduced in this book that are potentially of benefit in this manner are listed below:

1. Thirst, dry mouth[1]
- Bupleurum, Cinnamon Twig and Dried Ginger Decoction
- Eight-Ingredient Rehmannia Pills
- Ginseng Decoction
- Perfect Major Supplementation Decoction
- Poria Five Powder

2. Dysuria
- Achyranthes and Plantago Kidney Qi Pills
- Eight-Ingredient Rehmannia Pills
- Fangji and Astragalus Decoction
- Poria Five Powder

3. Menstrual disorders
- Blood-stasis formulas

4. Tremor
- Bupleurum, Cinnamon Twig and Dried Ginger Decoction
- Bupleurum Decoction Plus Dragon Bone and Oyster Shell
- Cinnamon Twig Decoction Plus Dragon Bone and Oyster Shell
- Liver-Repressing Powder Plus Tangerine Peel and Pinellia
- Uncaria Powder

5. Dizziness
- Coptis Toxin-Resolving Decoction
- String of Pearls Beverage
- Pinellia, Ovate Atractylodes and Gastrodia Decoction
- Poria, Cinnamon Twig, Ovate Atractylodes and Licorice Decoction
- Poria Five Powder
- Supplemented Free Wanderer Powder

---

[1] *White Tiger Plus Ginseng Decoction and Bupleurum and Poria Decoction, two formulas not introduced in this manual, have been found to be effective for drug-induced thirst in a small number of studies.*

6. Headaches
- Evodia Decoction
- Poria Five Powder
- Pueraria Decoction
- Uncaria Powder
- Other formulas for headaches introduced in the next chapter

7. Constipation[2]
- Freeing Abduction Powder
- Peach Kernel Qi-Infusing Decoction
- Supplemented Free Wanderer Powder
- Three Yellows Heart-Draining Decoction
- Other formulas containing rhubarb

8. Liver disorders
- Formulas containing bupleurum[3]
- Cinnamon Twig and Poria Pills
- Other blood stasis formulas[4]

As always, selection of remedies should be based on the overall symptom picture. Equally important, Kampo should not be used this way merely to enhance the palatability of drugs. Continued administration of the drugs in question should be a justifiable decision arrived at after careful deliberation.

Self-help measures for the patient

Alcohol, sedatives, and most psychedelic drugs are depressants, but are often used in self-treatment of depression. Patients with symptoms of depression should be cautioned that abuse of such substances can only worsen the problem.

---

[2] *Rhubarb and Licorice Decoction is a simple laxative formula having broad applicability in individuals of intermediate constitution. Intestine-Moistening Decoction is a gentle laxative remedy with lubricating and moisturizing actions frequently suitable for the asthenic in general and the elderly in particular.*

[3] *The Kampo formula most widely used for liver disorders is Minor Bupleurum Decoction.*

[4] *Blood stasis formulas are often combined with bupleurum flormulas in the treatment of liver disorders.*

EMOTIONAL DISTRESS

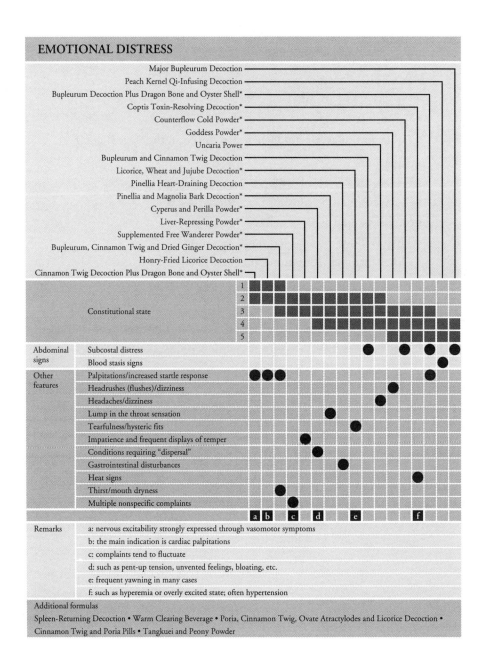

Major Bupleurum Decoction
Peach Kernel Qi-Infusing Decoction
Bupleurum Decoction Plus Dragon Bone and Oyster Shell*
Coptis Toxin-Resolving Decoction*
Counterflow Cold Powder*
Goddess Powder*
Uncaria Power
Bupleurum and Cinnamon Twig Decoction
Licorice, Wheat and Jujube Decoction*
Pinellia Heart-Draining Decoction
Pinellia and Magnolia Bark Decoction*
Cyperus and Perilla Powder*
Liver-Repressing Powder*
Supplemented Free Wanderer Powder*
Bupleurum, Cinnamon Twig and Dried Ginger Decoction*
Honry-Fried Licorice Decoction
Cinnamon Twig Decoction Plus Dragon Bone and Oyster Shell*

Constitutional state: 1 2 3 4 5

Abdominal signs	Subcostal distress	
	Blood stasis signs	
Other features	Palpitations/increased startle response	
	Headrushes (flushes)/dizziness	
	Headaches/dizziness	
	Lump in the throat sensation	
	Tearfulness/hysteric fits	
	Impatience and frequent displays of temper	
	Conditions requiring "dispersal"	
	Gastrointestinal disturbances	
	Heat signs	
	Thirst/mouth dryness	
	Multiple nonspecific complaints	

a b c d e f

Remarks	
a: nervous excitability strongly expressed through vasomotor symptoms	
b: the main indication is cardiac palpitations	
c: complaints tend to fluctuate	
d: such as pent-up tension, unvented feelings, bloating, etc.	
e: frequent yawning in many cases	
f: such as hyperemia or overly excited state; often hypertension	

Additional formulas

Spleen-Returning Decoction • Warm Clearing Beverage • Poria, Cinnamon Twig, Ovate Atractylodes and Licorice Decoction • Cinnamon Twig and Poria Pills • Tangkuei and Peony Powder

Chapter 16
Chronic Headaches

Headaches can be a sign of serious illness. Headaches that worsen steadily or severe headaches that begin suddenly require careful investigation to rule out the possibilities of life-threatening diseases. The discussion set forth here pertains to the management of headaches that many women experience during the climacteric years. It is also more broadly applicable to chronic recurring headaches considered to be functional in nature.

Such chronic headaches often respond well to Kampo treatment. Even intractable cases that had persisted for ten to twenty years despite the usual regimen of analgesics, vasodilators, and sedatives can be laid to rest with appropriate Kampo remedies. To be sure, no one system of healing contains all the answers. Their commonplaceness notwithstanding, headaches can be exceedingly difficult to treat. Patients should be encouraged to try other modes of treatment if Kampo remedies fail to work.

Constitutional aspects

The majority of recurrent headaches are associated with other complaints that may relate to every system of the body. For instance, digestive disturbances frequently figure in the symptom picture. These may be secondary to the stress generated by the headaches, or iatrogenic in nature, consequent to the use of headache medications that have adverse effects upon the digestive system. In Kampo, digestive dysfunction is also considered a possible etiologic factor in headaches.

Other common symptoms accompanying headaches include nervous tension, insomnia, headrushes, circulatory disorders, stiffness of neck, back, and shoulders, and menstrual problems. Chronic headaches are apt to be treated symptomatically. They should always be considered in the light of the total pattern. Do not overlook seemingly nonspecific and peripheral symptoms such as thirst and cold extremities. They can be valuable clues to pattern identification.

If psychologic and stress-related factors appear to be prominent in the symptom picture, additional formulas introduced in the chapter on emotional distress may be considered.

Kampo treatment

There is no Kampo remedy with a nonspecific pain-abolishing action for all headaches, although many herbs incorporated into the formulas do possess demonstrable analgesic and sedative properties. Beyond mitigation of pain, Kampo therapy aims to normalize the homeostatic mechanisms of the body and paves the way to healing from within.

Used judiciously, Kampo formulas rarely cause adverse reactions. They may be of particular benefit to headache sufferers who, due to a history of liver disorders, blood diseases, or peptic ulcers, cannot tolerate the usual modern drugs. They are also a viable alternative to the usual prophylactic treatment for migraine, which must be continued over a long period of time and is associated with a number of undesirable effects.

A. Classification of headaches

The Kampo approach can be effective in all forms of chronic recurring headaches. Classification of headaches into vascular, tension, etc., does not constitute a basis for Kampo diagnosis and treatment. However, where a formula has been found useful in a particular type of headache, this information is included as a reference in the accompanying table and in Part IV.

B. Evaluation of treatment

Kampo treatment usually takes effect slower than modern drugs, although a remedy such as Evodia Decoction can be relatively fast-acting when taken for acute attacks.

In general, favorable changes are observed after one to two weeks of therapy. Even if a decrease in the frequency of headaches is not obtained at first, other elements in the symptom picture should show improvement.

C. Combination with conventional medication

Drugs for the control of headaches may be used in conjunction with Kampo remedies. When depression is clearly at the root of the headache, anti-depressants may also be incorporated. However, many drugs are known to have adverse effects on the GI tract. Their use runs counter to a major principle of Kampo treatment: that normalization or strengthening of digestive function is of paramount importance in the treatment of any illness. Overuse of drugs can actually increase frequency of headaches. Consequently, drugs should not be taken on a regular basis. As much as possible, reserve them for the purpose of pain control during acute attacks, and prescribe no more than the necessary minimum dosage.

Self-help measures for the patient

Coffee drinkers should be aware that the regular use of coffee could well be the cause of their vascular headaches.

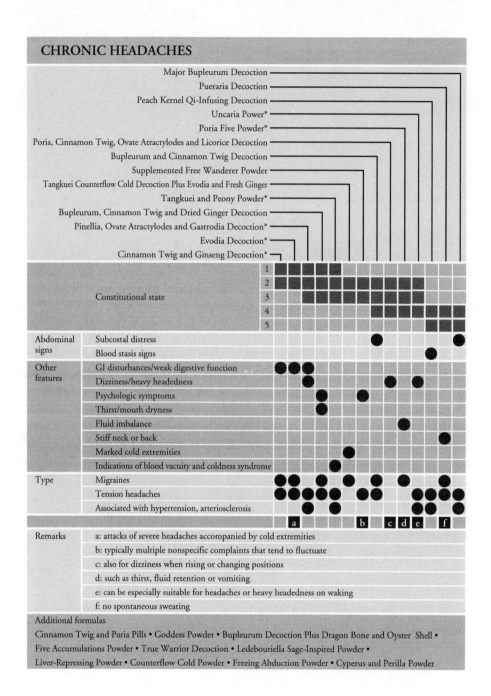

CHRONIC HEADACHES

Major Bupleurum Decoction
Pueraria Decoction
Peach Kernel Qi-Infusing Decoction
Uncaria Power*
Poria Five Powder*
Poria, Cinnamon Twig, Ovate Atractylodes and Licorice Decoction
Bupleurum and Cinnamon Twig Decoction
Supplemented Free Wanderer Powder
Tangkuei Counterflow Cold Decoction Plus Evodia and Fresh Ginger
Tangkuei and Peony Powder*
Bupleurum, Cinnamon Twig and Dried Ginger Decoction
Pinellia, Ovate Atractylodes and Gastrodia Decoction*
Evodia Decoction*
Cinnamon Twig and Ginseng Decoction*

	Constitutional state	1	
		2	
		3	
		4	
		5	
Abdominal signs	Subcostal distress		
	Blood stasis signs		
Other features	GI disturbances/weak digestive function		
	Dizziness/heavy headedness		
	Psychologic symptoms		
	Thirst/mouth dryness		
	Fluid imbalance		
	Stiff neck or back		
	Marked cold extremities		
	Indications of blood vacuity and coldness syndrome		
Type	Migraines		
	Tension headaches		
	Associated with hypertension, arteriosclerosis		

Remarks

a: attacks of severe headaches accompanied by cold extremities

b: typically multiple nonspecific complaints that tend to fluctuate

c: also for dizziness when rising or changing positions

d: such as thirst, fluid retention or vomiting

e: can be especially suitable for headaches or heavy headedness on waking

f: no spontaneous sweating

Additional formulas

Cinnamon Twig and Poria Pills • Goddess Powder • Bupleurum Decoction Plus Dragon Bone and Oyster Shell •
Five Accumulations Powder • True Warrior Decoction • Ledebouriella Sage-Inspired Powder •
Liver-Repressing Powder • Counterflow Cold Powder • Freeing Abduction Powder • Cyperus and Perilla Powder

Chapter 17
Abnormal Bleeding,
Vaginal Symptoms

I. Disturbances in menstrual pattern: Dysfunctional uterine bleeding

During the variable transitional phase before menopause, menstrual distur-bances are common and not necessarily a sign for concern. However, bleeding that is excessive, prolonged, or overly frequent requires investi-gation and treatment.

The problem is likely to be dysfunctional uterine bleeding (DUB) due to spo-radic ovulation in the premenopause.(2) This should not be assumed on the basis of the patient's age. Medical examination is essential to rule out specific organic causes (including benign lesions such as fibroids, polyps, endometriosis; inflam-matory processes such as endometritis and vaginitis; pelvic malignancies; and unexpected pregnancy). Appropriate medical or surgical intervention should be undertaken where necessary.

Kampo treatment

In treating DUB, the immediate objective is to halt the episode of prolonged or excessive bleeding that prompted the patient to seek care. Kampo treatment is usually adequate in this regard, but medical management is preferable if bleeding is profuse.

Once bleeding has stopped, Kampo can speed the recovery of patients who are anemic and weakened from bleeding. It can also be administered over a longer time span with the objective of preventing the recurrence of DUB in women of all ages. Judicious Kampo treatment may be expected to raise the general level of health and favor a climacteric with overall minimal discomfort. It is a viable option for women who desire an alternative to conventional measures or respond poorly to them.

Many remedies applicable in DUB appear to have a normalizing effect on the hypothalamic-pituitary-ovarian axis. These same remedies have been used with success in irregular menstruation, amenorrhea, infertility arising from a functional cause, premenstrual syndrome, and dysmenorrhea. Aspects of their mechanisms of action are beginning to be elucidated. For example, in vitro experiments have demonstrated that Channel-Warming Decoction acts on the hypothalamus and the pituitary to stimulate the secretion of gonadotropins; and that Tangkuei and Peony Powder stimulates pituitary secretion of gonadotropins and increases the production of progesterone by the corpus luteum. The usefulness of both remedies in the treatment of ovulatory dysfunction have been confirmed in preliminary clinical studies.(10)

Ligusticum, Tangkuei, Ass Hide Glue and Mugwort Decoction is the most widely applicable formula in DUB, either alone or in combination with other formulas. If hot flushes are a concomitant problem, several of the remedies listed in the accompanying table potentially alleviate both conditions.

A. Evaluation

Kampo remedies used to treat a non-profuse abnormal bleeding episode should stop the bleeding within one to several days. If bleeding does not cease within one week, even though the loss of blood is relatively small, other remedies or alternative measures should be tried.

In long-term treatment to prevent recurrence of abnormal bleeding, improvement of other aspects of the symptom picture is usually observable before assessment about DUB per se can be made, and generally signals the aptness of therapy. The subsequent menstrual pattern depends on individual factors, but Kampo therapy appears to favor a gradual decrease of menstruation in premenopausal women.

II. Postmenopausal bleeding

Any bleeding occurring nine months after menopause, including bloody discharge or spotting, requires careful investigation to rule out the possibility of malignancies.(8b) If the bleeding is found to be due to a benign cause such as atrophic vaginitis (see below), which accounts for 15% of all postmenopausal bleeding (8c), Kampo treatment can be very useful both in improving general health and the local condition of the lower genital tract.

III. Vaginal symptoms: Abnormal vaginal discharge, vaginal irritation, vaginitis

Symptoms of abnormal discharge, irritation in the genital area, and sometimes also urinary frequency and burning sensation upon urination can be due to infections by specific pathogens such as candida and trichomonas. Similar symptoms can be produced by nonspecific bacteria that are part of the vaginal and perineal flora, which can proliferate unchecked for a variety of reasons. Spermicidal creams and chemicals in vaginal douches and bath products can also induce such irritative reactions.

In menopausal women, gradual atrophic changes occur in many body structures consequent to aging and reduced estrogen production. Atrophy also affects the lower vaginal tract. The mucosa of the vagina thins progressively, loses elasticity, becomes more fragile, and produces less secretions. The amount of lubrication produced during sexual activity diminishes as well as the speed with which it is produced. The vaginal environment becomes less acidic, even alkaline, allowing the growth of many bacterial pathogens.(4,11)

As a result, the vagina can become prone to inflammations and infections in older women. Atrophic vaginitis can develop, a chronic nonspecific inflammation causing watery discharge, itching or burning, spotting, and often also irritative urinary symptoms. Sometimes vaginitis due to specific infection may be superimposed on atrophic vaginitis. Women may also experience frictional dyspareunia because of insufficient lubrication, possibly with spotting or bleeding due to tearing of the vaginal tissue during intercourse. Moreover, the elevated vaginal pH means that the buffering capacity of the vagina against the alkaline semen is lowered. Intercourse can therefore produce burning.(8c)

Degenerative changes in the external genitalia usually do not give rise to significant symptoms until some years past menopause. Although inevitable, they apparently may be delayed. Regular sexual activity helps keep the vagina elastic and lubricated, and can possibly stave off the onset of atrophy for many years.(7)

Conventional treatment

Gynecologic examinations are mandatory. Modern medications generally works well in abolishing acute inflammations of the genitals due to infections. Since they upset the balance of protective flora and tend to diminish host resistance, they are not recommended in chronic or recurrent cases.

As for degenerative changes, estrogen therapy has been shown to be effective both in relief of symptoms and reversal of atrophy. However, the problem often recurs when estrogen is discontinued.(1)

Kampo treatment

Kampo treatment may be very effective for abnormal vaginal discharge and vaginal irritation. Though most of the remedies employed contain substances with anti-inflammatory, bacteriocidal, and possibly estrogenic actions, they are weak compared to drugs. Kampo apparently also works through constitutional improvement, promoting circulation in the pelvis and the genital area, enhancing the natural self-cleaning action of the vagina and fostering a protective vaginal flora.

For acute infections, sthenically-oriented formulas that are stronger in anti-inflammatory action may be used for short term in all except markedly asthenic patients. Watch for adverse reactions such as digestive disturbance. If diarrhea occurs, it should not be allowed to persist too long or to debilitate the patient. While not a therapeutic option in modern medicine, some purgation is desirable to aid in the detoxification and lessening of inflammation.

Within the framework of modern medicine, Kampo is perhaps most valuable in chronic or recurrent vaginitis, atrophic and otherwise. It can also be tried for vaginal symptoms not associated with any discernible organic changes.

A. Evaluation

Improvement in subjective symptoms is often obtained within two weeks of treatment. If urinary frequency and burning on urination are related to the vaginal problems, these will also be relieved by Kampo therapy.

B. Combination with conventional medication

For acute cases, the most desirable strategy may be to maximize therapeutic benefit by combining Kampo with modern drugs. Drugs may be given alone or supplemented with a Kampo remedy for quick control of acute symptoms, then Kampo treatment may be continued to foster true recovery and prevent recurrence. This applies also to estrogen therapy. A short course of estrogen may be given to relieve symptoms of severe atrophy. Then it may be replaced by Kampo.

IV. A note on premenstrual syndrome

As noted previously, many of the formulas can benefit various problems related to the menstrual cycle, including premenstrual syndrome (PMS).

Many women experience a worsening of PMS during the premenopausal phase. Though the cyclic premenstrual symptoms usually end with menopause, they may persist for some years afterwards, occasionally into the 6th decade. PMS actually begins with the onset of natural menopause in about 10% of sufferers. Artificial menopause (from hysterectomy and/or oophorectomy) may increase the severity of pre-existing PMS, and may even initiate it. Thus, neither menstruation nor the presence of uterus and ovaries appears to be necessary for the occurrence of PMS.(12)

While some clinicians speculate that PMS is a problem of the early climacteric, the relationship between menopause and PMS is not clear. It has been observed that menopausal women who have experienced more intense PMS require higher dosages of hormone to control their symptoms. Hot flushes and chills, the hallmarks of climacteric syndrome, can occur in some women suffering from moderate to severe PMS. There is in fact a considerable overlap in symptomatology. Without careful monthly charting to reveal their cyclic nature, premenstrual symptoms may be erroneously attributed to climacteric syndrome.

It is perhaps more than incidental that the very same acronym can be formed from premenstrual syndrome and perimenopausal symptoms: The molecular mechanisms responsible for the two may well be identical in some respects. Clinicians will appreciate the fact that, as long as the pattern of symptoms matches the prescribing criteria, the same Kampo remedy may be employed to alleviate either PMS or climacteric complaints.

ABNORMAL BLEEDING • MENSTRUAL DISORDERS • VAGINAL SYMPTOMS

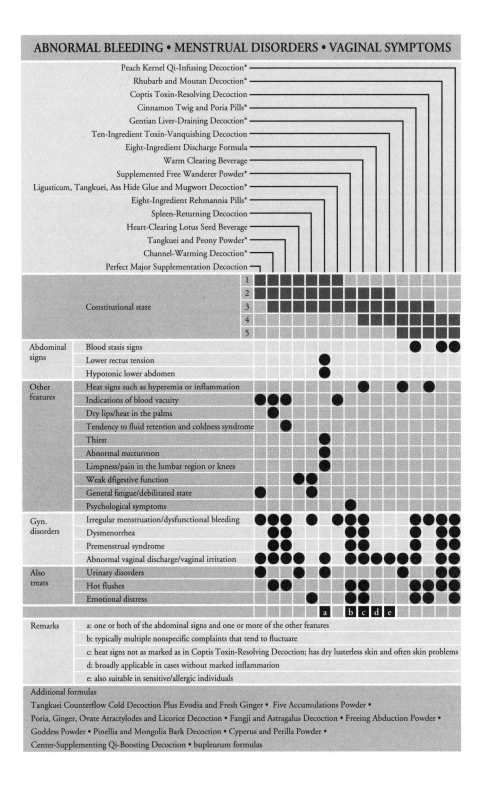

Formulas (listed across the top of the chart):

- Peach Kernel Qi-Infusing Decoction*
- Rhubarb and Moutan Decoction*
- Coptis Toxin-Resolving Decoction
- Cinnamon Twig and Poria Pills*
- Gentian Liver-Draining Decoction*
- Ten-Ingredient Toxin-Vanquishing Decoction
- Eight-Ingredient Discharge Formula
- Warm Clearing Beverage
- Supplemented Free Wanderer Powder*
- Ligusticum, Tangkuei, Ass Hide Glue and Mugwort Decoction*
- Eight-Ingredient Rehmannia Pills*
- Spleen-Returning Decoction
- Heart-Clearing Lotus Seed Beverage
- Tangkuei and Peony Powder*
- Channel-Warming Decoction*
- Perfect Major Supplementation Decoction

Constitutional state: 1 2 3 4 5

Abdominal signs	Blood stasis signs
	Lower rectus tension
	Hypotonic lower abdomen
Other features	Heat signs such as hyperemia or inflammation
	Indications of blood vacuity
	Dry lips/heat in the palms
	Tendency to fluid retention and coldness syndrome
	Thirst
	Abnormal micturition
	Limpness/pain in the lumbar region or knees
	Weak dfigestive function
	General fatigue/debilitated state
	Psychological symptoms
Gyn. disorders	Irregular menstruation/dysfunctional bleeding
	Dysmenorrhea
	Premenstrual syndrome
	Abnormal vaginal discharge/vaginal irritation
Also treats	Urinary disorders
	Hot flushes
	Emotional distress

a b c d e

Remarks

a: one or both of the abdominal signs and one or more of the other features

b: typically multiple nonspecific complaints that tend to fluctuate

c: heat signs not as marked as in Coptis Toxin-Resolving Decoction; has dry lusterless skin and often skin problems

d: broadly applicable in cases without marked inflammation

e: also suitable in sensitive/allergic individuals

Additional formulas

Tangkuei Counterflow Cold Decoction Plus Evodia and Fresh Ginger • Five Accumulations Powder •
Poria, Ginger, Ovate Atractylodes and Licorice Decoction • Fangji and Astragalus Decoction • Freeing Abduction Powder •
Goddess Powder • Pinellia and Mongolia Bark Decoction • Cyperus and Perilla Powder •
Center-Supplementing Qi-Boosting Decoction • bupleurum formulas

Chapter 18
Urinary Disorders

This chapter addresses certain lower urinary tract problems that tend to affect climacteric women. It is not meant to be a comprehensive treatment guideline on urinary disorders.

Lower urinary tract problems are very common in women. Treatment with antibiotics can quickly clear symptoms due to an acute bacterial infection. But infection recurs in many cases and becomes a scourge for patient and physician alike. Sometimes, the clinical presentation mimics bacterial cystitis, yet no causative disease process can be discovered. Termed "urethral syndrome," this condition is seen primarily in middle-aged women who may or may not have a history of urinary infections. It is characterized by frequency, urgency, and dysuria in the absence of bacteriuria; and sometimes also pyuria (the presence of pus in the urine). Tension and anxiety are believed to contribute to its etiology. Conventional treatment is usually ineffective in such instances.(13a)

The lower urinary tract and the lower genital tract are in close proximity and have the same embryonic origin. Lower urinary tract disorders may be closely related to lower genital tract disorders, and vice versa. Vaginitis, for example, often produces some cystitis-like signs and symptoms. In postmenopausal women, an elevated pH of vaginal secretions permits the proliferation of pathogenic bacteria in the perineal area, which can become the source of recurrent cystitis.(14)

In the later climacteric, atrophic changes also affect the epithelium of the urethra and the bladder trigone. Weakness of urethral sphincter function can develop. The pelvic floor musculature, which may have been weakened or damaged earlier due to childbirth and other factors, further loses strength and elasticity. These alterations may lead to urgency, urethral syndrome, and incontinence.(4,11)

Incontinence is among the most distressing urinary disorders. It can gravely limit the social and private activities of women. Usually a problem endured in private, it is a source of considerable inconvenience and psychological burden to the patient even if only a small amount is lost.(11,15) Stress incontinence is the most common form, followed by urge incontinence associated with detrusor instability (also termed unstable bladder or irritable bladder).(13b)

Often the onset of incontinence or exacerbation of existing symptoms is related to menopause.(15) Weak pelvic muscles and urethral atrophy are only some of the more obvious parameters. Continence depends on the proper working of many delicate mechanisms. Subtle functional abnormalities that are both difficult to diagnose and treat may be involved.

Kampo treatment

1. Infections

Compared to men, women have a shorter urethra and are more vulnerable to the entry of bacteria into the urinary tract. Yet a bacterial invasion does not easily become established as an infection in healthy individuals. Repeated infections suggest a weakness in the immune system. Rather than regarding the body as the battleground between bacteria and drugs, Kampo takes a constitutional approach. Treatment stimulates and support the body's inherent defense functions in addition to relief of distressing symptoms.

Mild to moderate cases of bacterial infection can often be treated with Kampo remedies alone. However, to ensure quick control of infections, antibiotics are best combined in the acute stage. In recurrent infections, long-term therapy is desirable to improve general health and correct underlying tendencies to infections, and thereby lessen relapses that often plague modern drug therapy.

2. Urethral syndrome

Urethral syndrome and other urinary problems in which subjective complaints far exceed urologic findings baffles conventional management, since they have poorly defined etiology and pathogenesis. A wholistic assessment is especially pertinent here. The Kampo strategy of balance and nurture can help bring about improvement in both the somatic and psychological aspects of such disorders.

3. Incontinence

Kampo therapy emphasizes raising the overall level of vitality. It is well worth a try where conventional measures have proven ineffective. Even if no significant improvement results in incontinence per se, such therapy is meaningful in that it increases the physical and mental reserve of the patient who must live with this difficult problem.

4. Atrophic changes

As always, treatment is based on a consideration of the entire symptom picture. Proper diagnosis should lead to selection of a formula that will also address the factor of atrophy.

5. Other urinary problems

In addition to the conditions discussed above, Kampo therapy is well worth a try in all chronic urinary disorders not amenable to conventional pharmacotherapy or surgery. It can possibly improve subjective symptoms and the quality of life even in cases with dismal outlook.

A. Remedies

The most widely applied formula for the alleviation of symptoms in the acute stage is perhaps Polyporus Decoction. It is often combined with antibiotics in the treatment of bacterial infections.

As indicated in the accompanying table, some remedies for urinary disorders also treat concomitant vaginal discharge, pain, and itching. Since lower genital tract problems are often implicated in urinary disturbances, other remedies that appear in the table for abnormal bleeding/vaginal symptoms may also be pertinent. In particular, Supplemented Free Wanderer Powder, Tangkuei and Peony Powder, or Cinnamon Twig and Poria Pills each by itself may be adequate for mild nonspecific urinary symptoms associated with climacteric syndrome.

Circulatory impairment is a contributing factor in various lower urinary tract disorders. The three formulas named above belong to the category of blood stasis-dispelling remedies, and have in common the specific property of promoting circulation in the pelvis and urogenital areas. Improved circulation enhances the immune mechanisms, helps to reverse degenerative changes in the musculature and epithelial tissues, and may be very beneficial in restoring proper bladder and urethral functions.

Coldness is apt to be overlooked in biomedicine, yet it can be an important etiologic or exacerbating factor in urinary problems. Kampo is particularly useful where the symptom picture includes features of coldness. Remedies such as Tangkuei and Peony Powder and Poria, Ginger, Ovate Atractylodes and Licorice Decoction owe their effectiveness in part to a warming effect on the lower body.

In cases of incontinence, modern urological classification does not necessarily guide the selection of formulas. Such formulas as Eight-Ingredient Rehmannia Pills and Heart-Clearing Lotus Seed Beverage may be applicable in all forms. A constitutional approach is advised rather than a narrow focus on the incontinence. More specifically, incontinence associated with poor muscle tone or decline in function is perceived in Kampo as an asthenic state. Remedies with tonic and nutritive effects, such as Center-Supplementing Qi-Boosting Decoction and Perfect Major Supplementation Decoction can be beneficial. Incontinence associated with urgency (as in detrusor instability) and other irritative symptoms may respond to formulas useful in cystourethritis/urethral syndrome. Examples are Polyporus Decoction, Gentian Liver-Draining Decoction, and Five Stranguries Powder.

Stress and anxiety also affect urinary function. Remedies such as Pinellia and Magnolia Bark Decoction or Bupleurum Decoction Plus Dragon Bone and Oyster Shell may be beneficial in cases featuring prominent pychological elements (refer to the Emotional Distress table).

Peony and Licorice Decoction can be administered adjunctively to help alleviate painful spasms and marked dysuria.

B. Evaluation

Usually, one to three days will be required to settle acute symptoms of an infection, although prompt treatment with an appropriate remedy can bring relief within half a day. One week should be sufficient to evaluate the effectiveness of the prescribed remedy or combination of remedies. In patients susceptible to repeated episodes of infection, treatment (possibly involving a change of prescription) should be continued for one to several months after the symptoms disappear.

Chronic problems in general require long-term treatment. Prognosis depends on the nature of the disorder and the constitutional condition of the patient. When the response is favorable, significant improvement is seen after 2-4 weeks of therapy, and resolution may be obtained within 3-6 months.

C. Combination with conventional medication

When antibiotics and other drugs are employed for acute urinary infections, conjunctive Kampo therapy is recommended both to shorten the course of drug use and to treat the symptoms that may remain after the disappearance of pathogens from the urine: frequency, dysuria, feeling of incomplete voiding, lower abdominal pain, etc. Kampo can also be administered after a course of drugs to treat lingering symptoms.

If estrogen is prescribed for irritative symptoms related to urethral atrophy in the later climacteric, Kampo therapy may be combined to allow for gradual reduction and eventual discontinuance of the hormone.

The same consideration applies for estrogen and other types of drugs given to treat the various forms of incontinence, and Kampo can certainly be utilized to aid recovery from surgical repair.

Self-help measures for the patient

• Pelvic floor exercises may be performed to help prevent or relieve symptoms associated with tissue weakness (incontinence, difficulty emptying the bladder). A number of self-help books describe these exercises in detail.

• Avoid caffeine, alcohol, and tobacco. All are irritants of the urinary system.

URINARY DISORDERS

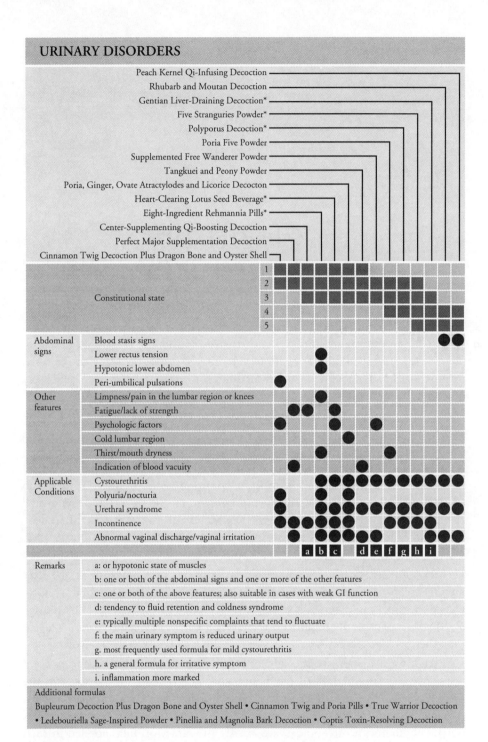

Formulas (listed across the top):
- Peach Kernel Qi-Infusing Decoction
- Rhubarb and Moutan Decoction
- Gentian Liver-Draining Decoction*
- Five Stranguries Powder*
- Polyporus Decoction*
- Poria Five Powder
- Supplemented Free Wanderer Powder
- Tangkuei and Peony Powder
- Poria, Ginger, Ovate Atractylodes and Licorice Decocton
- Heart-Clearing Lotus Seed Beverage*
- Eight-Ingredient Rehmannia Pills*
- Center-Supplementing Qi-Boosting Decoction
- Perfect Major Supplementation Decoction
- Cinnamon Twig Decoction Plus Dragon Bone and Oyster Shell

	Constitutional state (1–5)
Abdominal signs	Blood stasis signs
	Lower rectus tension
	Hypotonic lower abdomen
	Peri-umbilical pulsations
Other features	Limpness/pain in the lumbar region or knees
	Fatigue/lack of strength
	Psychologic factors
	Cold lumbar region
	Thirst/mouth dryness
	Indication of blood vacuity
Applicable Conditions	Cystourethritis
	Polyuria/nocturia
	Urethral syndrome
	Incontinence
	Abnormal vaginal discharge/vaginal irritation

Remarks

a: or hypotonic state of muscles

b: one or both of the abdominal signs and one or more of the other features

c: one or both of the above features; also suitable in cases with weak GI function

d: tendency to fluid retention and coldness syndrome

e: typically multiple nonspecific complaints that tend to fluctuate

f: the main urinary symptom is reduced urinary output

g. most frequently used formula for mild cystourethritis

h. a general formula for irritative symptom

i. inflammation more marked

Additional formulas

Bupleurum Decoction Plus Dragon Bone and Oyster Shell • Cinnamon Twig and Poria Pills • True Warrior Decoction • Ledebouriella Sage-Inspired Powder • Pinellia and Magnolia Bark Decoction • Coptis Toxin-Resolving Decoction

Chapter 19
Body Aches and Pains

Muscle and joint pains in perimenopausal women are among the scores of symptoms associated with the diminishment of ovarian function. Medical dictionaries even identify a type of arthritis (termed menopausal or climacteric arthritis) attributed to ovarian hormonal deficiency that affects the small joints, shoulders, elbows, or knees.

Some common joint and muscle diseases tend to develop at this time of life or affect women disproportionately. Osteoarthritis, which results from wear and tear on the joints, evolves in middle age and is prevalent in people over 60. It is the most common type of arthritis, and its severe form affects three times as many women as men. Rheumatoid arthritis, a common autoimmune disorder, also afflicts two to three times more women than men. Fibrositis, a clinical syndrome characterized by chronic pain and stiffness of muscles in the neck, shoulders, back, and other sites, manifests mostly in women in the fourth to fifth decade.[1] There is usually no detectable organic cause.

Osteoporosis, a significant problem among non-black women after menopause, is perhaps the most pertinent example. The risk of vertebral fractures related to spinal osteoporosis is estimated to be 25% in white women by the age of 50 years.[1] Symptomatic spinal osteoporosis, which may cause chronic pain in the lower back or extremities, occurs in five times as many women as men.[2]

Except for osteoporosis, the subject of the next chapter, the conditions cited above have no specific link to the menopause. It is not within the scope of the present manual to consider them in detail. However, body aches and pains are a rather common experience of women in the climacteric, and many formulas potentially useful in osteoporosis are exactly the same formulas applied in such

---

[1] *Also known as myofascial pain syndrome, primary fibromyalgia syndrome, psychogenic rheumatism, and several other terms. The profusion of diagnostic labels reflect the lack of knowledge regarding its etiology and pathology.*

disorders. In order to maximize both the utility of these formulas and the ability of the practitioner to meet the demands of women in this stage of life, treatment guidelines broadly applicable in common musculoskeletal conditions are provided in this chapter.

Traditional concepts

Osteoarthrits, rheumatoid arthritis, sciatica, etc. are distinct entities in modern medicine. However, many of the outward manifestations are similar, as reflected in the common use of analgesics and anti-inflammatory drugs for symptomatic relief in these disorders. From the Kampo point of view, the signs and symptoms shared by painful disorders of joints and soft tissues can be conceptualized in terms of blood imbalance, fluid imbalance, cold, and heat. Fluid imbalance here refers in particular to symptoms of stagnation such as joint effusion, stiffness, and edema. Fluid stagnation is said to be predisposed or exacerbated by cold and damp, consistent with the well-known phenomenon that rheumatic symptoms tend to be worse in cold, damp weather.

Heat is exemplified by the rubor and warmth of joint inflammations. Cold, which tends to predominate in chronic cases, refers both to the etiology and the nature of symptoms. In the former sense, it is generally linked with wind and damp as environmental influences contributing to the pathogenesis and aggravation of painful symptoms. In the latter sense, it refers to coldness symptoms experienced by the patient.

Kampo treatment

The progression of musculoskeletal afflictions can vary greatly from person to person, demanding attention to individual factors. Chronic cases often have ramifications throughout the entire body and are best approached systemically. Conventional management stresses identification and treatment of the underlying cause. Yet often the underlying mechanism of painful symptoms is obscure or cannot be treated. Modern pharmacotherapy is then limited to symptomatic relief and may need to be continued indefinitely. The analgesic, anti-inflammatory, and other drugs used for this purpose are associated with a variety of adverse effects, often cumulative in nature.

Such considerations bespeak a role for Kampo in this field of medicine. The usual statements may be made regarding its special applicability in persons with digestive impairment and the elderly. In addition, the warming action of many Kampo remedies is particularly beneficial in cases with significant coldness symptoms.

Although substances having demonstrable analgesic, antispasmodic, anti-inflammatory, diuretic, diaphoretic, or peripheral vasodilatory properties are incorporated in Kampo formulas used for rheumatism, they are weak relative to modern drugs for the most part, and do not wholly account for the therapeutic benefits of the formulas. In fact, the analgesic effect of a given remedy may vary considerably from patient to patient, suggesting that synergy of component substances and host factors may be operative. If relief of pain is all that is desired, modern drugs are faster and surer acting. As noted below, the two modes of treatment may be combined to advantage.

Common formulas for rheumatic conditions are listed in the accompanying table. While examples of applicable disorders are also indicated, it must be emphasized that the basis for selection of appropriate remedy is the pattern, not the particular disease entity. As long as the same pattern is diagnosed, the same formula may be used to treat osteoarthritis, rheumatoid arthritis, sciatica, or any other disorders producing similar symptoms.

Minor body aches and pains accompanying hot flushes in the perimenopause may subside after treatment with Kampo remedies applicable in hot flushes, which include some formulas beneficial for joint and muscle pains. Depending on concurrent disorders, formulas introduced in other chapters may also be relevant.

A. Remedies

Formulas containing ephedra tend to be suitable during acute to subacute stages. Examples from the table are Spleen-Effusing Decoction Plus Ovate Atractylodes and Pueraria Decoction. They can also be used during the chronic stages (possibly as adjuncts to other formulas) if indications exist. In the elderly and other asthenic persons, ephedra formulas should be applied with caution and are best commenced at a reduced dosage. Formulas suitable for chronic administration often incorporate aconite, tangkuei, and fangji. Examples are Cinnamon Twig Decoction Plus Atractylodes and Aconite, Channel-Coursing Blood-Quickening Decoction, and Fangji and Astragalus Decoction.

A remedy may be considered from the standpoint of its cooling or warming effects. Spleen-Effusing Decoction Plus Ovate Atractylodes typifies the former, and Cinnamon Twig Decoction Plus Atractylodes and Aconite the latter. In order to match the particular mixture of cold and heat characteristics in a given case, the need may arise clinically to combine available formula extracts or add extracts of single substances. A common example is the use of extra aconite to augment the warming and analgesic effects of a base formula (see below, Additions). Another common practice is to mix Spleen-Effusing Decotion Plus Ovate Atractylodes (an ephedra formula) with a coldness- and asthenia-oriented formula (such as Cinnamon Twig Decoction Plus Atractylodes and Aconite, or Fangji and Astragalus Decoction) to treat local heat and swelling in a predominately cold pattern. The proportion should be adjusted as necessary.

Spleen-Effusing Decoction Plus Ovate Atractylodes, Coix Decoction, and Cinnamon Twig Decoction Plus Atractylodes and Aconite are formulated largely for the purpose of symptom relief. Clinically, it may be necessary to fortify the effects of such remedies on constitutional factors, especially in chronic cases. Three general categories of formulas that are often useful in this manner are blood stasis formulas, bupleurum formulas, and formulas that normalize the GI function and/or increase the level of overall health.

Peony and Licorice Decoction may be prescribed as an adjunct to other formulas on an as-needed basis for relief of painful spasms or marked pain accompanying flexing of joints.

In chronic cases featuring a marked degree of generalized fatigue, blood vacuity, and impaired digestive function, the therapeutic priority may be to first build up overall health with a formula such as Perfect Major Supplementation Decoction, Center-Supplementing Qi-Boosting Decoction, Six Gentlemen Decoction, or Spleen-Returning Decoction, introduced in the chapter on osteoporosis and elsewhere in the book.

B. Additions

Adding aconite to a base formula will augment the effectiveness if indications exist, i.e., for marked coldness or pain that worsens with cold stimuli. The dosage may be increased gradually for persistent pain and coldness. Aconite (in an aconite-containing formula or as a supplement) is not suitable if it leads to increased pain. Consider blood stasis remedies instead, especially the ones formulated with tangkuei. Extra ginseng, rhubarb, etc., may also be desirable in a given case. Please refer to Chapter 10 for information regarding addition of aconite and rhubarb.

C. Evaluation

As a rule, the more chronic the case, the slower the improvement is likely to be. Nevertheless, at least some signs of contitutional improvement should be observable following two to four weeks of treatment.

Additional notes pertaining to arthritis, chronic low back pain/sciatica, and fibrositis are provided below.

Arthritis (osteoarthritis, rheumatoid arthritis [RA], etc).

An appropriate remedy or combination of remedies taken over time can help to retard progression of these diseases.

In all but mild cases of RA, Kampo therapy is best applied in the context of a larger treatment program involving biomedical management. It can be very useful in treating constitutional factors or concurrent conditions that may exacerbate RA. The duration of morning stiffness, being one of the most sensitive clinical parameters of the disease activity, may be used to assess the therapeutic effectiveness.

Fangji and Astragalus Decoction (possibly in combination with Spleen-Effusing Decoction Plus Ovate Atractylodes) and Coix Decoction are frequently applied in osteoarthritis of the knee. A suitable blood stasis formula may be added if there is fatigue or pain in the legs, varicose veins, or other indications of circulatory impairment.

Chronic low back pain/sciatica

Blood stasis formulas are often beneficial in chronic low back pain, especially in cases related to gynecologic disorders. Cinnamon Twig and Poria Pills, Peach Kernel Qi-Infusing Decoction, and Freeing Abduction Powder are also suitable for acute backache or sciatica from injury, even in the absence of abdominal blood stasis signs. They may cause diarrhea, which is harmless for a few days as long as it does not weaken the patient. Purging can actually aid in quick recovery from injuries, and additional rhubarb may be added for this purpose.

Eight-Ingredient Rehmannia Pills is a formula frequently suitable for older patients, and also where diabetes or urinary disorders are implicated. Bupleurum formulas may be appropriate in cases with subcostal distress.

Sciatica shares with other neuralgias the peculiarity that the more severe the pain, the faster it will heal. Milder cases are actually harder to treat. With modern treatment, sciatica can last from a few days to several weeks or more, and it tends to recur. In contrast, sciatica that responds well to Kampo remedies is often completely cured.

Fibrositis

Like many rheumatic conditions, fibrositis tend to be worse in cold and damp weather. Kampo treatment may be effective in relieving the symptoms and preventing recurrence of attacks. In addition to formulas indicated in the table, remedies for stiffness and pain in the neck and shoulder area include:

- Bupleurum formulas
- Uncaria Powder
- Pinellia, Ovate Atractylodes and Gastrodia Decoction
- Six Gentlemen Decoction

Use of acupuncture

The efficacy of acumoxa therapy in musculoskeletal disorders is well known. Properly applied, this therapy can shorten the period of healing. Often the concomitant use of Kampo and acupuncture has a mutually enhancing effect.

Combination with conventional treatment

Although it is possible to control relatively mild cases by Kampo alone, beyond a certain degree of severity and for purposes of quick symptom relief, most Kampo extracts are not as effective as modern nonsteroid anti-inflammatory drugs (NSAIDs), muscle relaxants, antirheumatic drugs, and immunosuppressant drugs. Moreover, the more advanced the organic change, the more need there is for modern medical intervention in general. Hence, the most practical approach in many cases is to optimize therapeutic potency and safety by adroitly combining Kampo and conventional measures.

A summary of possible strategies of combination therapy follows, together with some examples drawn from formulas introduced in this manual.

1. Use drugs to control acute episodes and Kampo as maintenance therapy to deal with milder symptoms and wider constitutional factors.
2. Reduce the dosage of drugs and thereby lower the likelihood of drug toxicity through parallel use of Kampo therapy.

3. Treat symptoms not relieved by drugs with Kampo.

4. Increase vigor in patients debilitated by chronic illness and chronic polypharmacy with Kampo remedies such as Center-Supplementing Qi-Boosting Decoction and Perfect Major Supplementation Decoction.

5. Use Kampo to counter side effects of drugs, so that the latter may be continued where justified.

   Bupleurum formulas, blood stasis formulas, and formulas containing ginseng as well as extra ginseng extract are frequently suitable in treating side effects of drugs. For example:

   • Indigestion, diarrhea, gastric ulcer, and other gastrointestinal problems are possible complications from the chronic use of NSAIDs. They may be lessened by use of such formulas as Bupleurum and Cinnamon Twig Decoction, Pinellia Heart-Draining Decoction, Six Gentlemen Decoction, Center-Supplementing Qi-Boosting Decoction, True Warrior Decoction, Ginseng Decoction, or Cinnamon Twig and Ginseng Decoction.

   • Hypertension, hyperlipidemia, and accelerated atherosclerosis associated with the use of corticosteroids may be countered by Major Bupleurum Decoction, Cinnamon Twig and Poria Pills, and other formulas applicable in hypertension.

6. Apply Kampo as a complement to physical and occupational therapies, exercises to strengthen muscles without straining the joints, traction, weight reduction, surgery, etc.

   Combining Kampo with such nonpharmacologic techniques may obviate drug use or limit it to occasional administration.

Combination therapy is by no means a self-evident issue. The exact treatment plan depends on the nature of disease, severity of symptoms, and individual circumstances. Therapeutic trials are necessary to find the most effective and least toxic combination regimen for a particular patient.

BODY ACHES AND PAINS

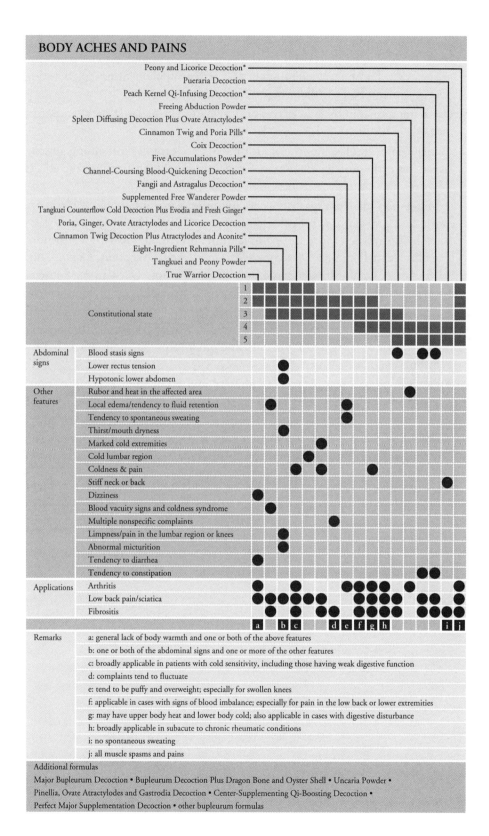

		True Warrior Decoction	Tangkuei and Peony Powder	Eight-Ingredient Rehmannia Pills*	Cinnamon Twig Decoction Plus Atractylodes and Aconite*	Poria, Ginger, Ovate Atractylodes and Licorice Decoction	Tangkuei Counterflow Cold Decoction Plus Evodia and Fresh Ginger*	Supplemented Free Wanderer Powder	Fangji and Astragalus Decoction*	Channel-Coursing Blood-Quickening Decoction*	Five Accumulations Powder*	Coix Decoction*	Cinnamon Twig and Poria Pills*	Spleen Diffusing Decoction Plus Ovate Atractylodes*	Freeing Abduction Powder	Peach Kernel Qi-Infusing Decoction*	Pueraria Decoction	Peony and Licorice Decoction*
Constitutional state	1	■	■	■	■	■												■
	2	■	■	■	■	■	■	■	■	■	■							■
	3		■	■	■	■	■	■	■	■	■	■	■					■
	4									■	■	■	■	■	■	■	■	■
	5												■	■	■	■	■	■
Abdominal signs	Blood stasis signs												●		●	●		
	Lower rectus tension			●														
	Hypotonic lower abdomen			●														
Other features	Rubor and heat in the affected area													●				
	Local edema/tendency to fluid retention		●						●									
	Tendency to spontaneous sweating								●									
	Thirst/mouth dryness			●														
	Marked cold extremities						●											
	Cold lumbar region					●												
	Coldness & pain				●		●				●							
	Stiff neck or back																●	
	Dizziness	●																
	Blood vacuity signs and coldness syndrome		●															
	Multiple nonspecific complaints							●										
	Limpness/pain in the lumbar region or knees			●														
	Abnormal micturition			●														
	Tendency to diarrhea	●																
	Tendency to constipation														●	●		
Applications	Arthritis	●			●				●	●	●	●		●				●
	Low back pain/sciatica	●	●	●	●	●	●			●	●	●	●		●	●		●
	Fibrositis		●		●		●	●		●	●	●	●		●	●	●	●
		a		b	c			d	e	f	g	h					i	j

Remarks

a: general lack of body warmth and one or both of the above features

b: one or both of the abdominal signs and one or more of the other features

c: broadly applicable in patients with cold sensitivity, including those having weak digestive function

d: complaints tend to fluctuate

e: tend to be puffy and overweight; especially for swollen knees

f: applicable in cases with signs of blood imbalance; especially for pain in the low back or lower extremities

g: may have upper body heat and lower body cold; also applicable in cases with digestive disturbance

h: broadly applicable in subacute to chronic rheumatic conditions

i: no spontaneous sweating

j: all muscle spasms and pains

Additional formulas

Major Bupleurum Decoction • Bupleurum Decoction Plus Dragon Bone and Oyster Shell • Uncaria Powder • Pinellia, Ovate Atractylodes and Gastrodia Decoction • Center-Supplementing Qi-Boosting Decoction • Perfect Major Supplementation Decoction • other bupleurum formulas

Chapter 20
Osteoporosis

Osteoporosis is a condition in which the bone has lost sufficient mass to sustain a fracture with minimal trauma. It affects 15 to 20 million Americans, and accounts for some 1.3 million fractures per year at an annual health care cost of $6 billion.(1) Both men and women lose bone mass as they age, but a period of rapid loss occurs in women with the onset of menopause. It has been estimated that nearly half of the women in the US over age 50 have some degree of osteoporosis.(3)

Overt symptoms are generally absent until a fracture occurs. Most typically, this takes the form of compression fracture of one or more vertebrae, which can result in progressive deformity, loss of height, and chronic pain. Two other common sites of fractures are the hip and the wrist. Hip fracture carries high morbidity and mortality rates and is the most serious complication of osteoporosis.

As is true for many other diseases, primary prophylactic measures for osteoporosis consist of proper nutrition, a sensible excercise program, and other good health habits practiced early on by the individual. Estrogen therapy combined with adequate calcium has been shown to retard bone loss and reduce risk of fractures in postmenopausal women. For estrogen to be an effective prophylaxis, it must be started before osteoporosis is established and must be continued indefinitely. Other available medical therapies include fluoride, calcitonin, and the anabolic steroids. Fluoride is still experimental and causes a considerable number of side effects, while the long-term safety and efficacy of synthetic calcitonin and anabolic steroids have yet to be demonstrated.(8d)

The quest for therapeutic methods with few adverse effects suitable for long-term administration has led some Japanese physicians to explore the use of Kampo in osteoporosis. Kampo medicine abounds in remedies for aging-related degenerative changes, including low back pain and other musculoskeletal problems in older people. However, osteoporosis might be said to number among its newer applications. It is unlikely to have been a significant phenomenon in the past when the average life span was shorter and sedentariness not a public health concern. The ancients also had no way of measuring bone density, even if they did observe that bones become more fragile with age. A Kampo physician would perceive osteoporosis indirectly, inferring the state of bone health from sensory information about the entire body. He or she would deal with osteoporosis the same way as with with any other disease: by identifying imbalances and attempting to restore balance, which in concrete terms means relieving symptoms and improving the constitutional condition.

Kampo treatment

Research on the use of Kampo to control the rate of bone loss only began recently and has concentrated on a small number of remedies. Thus far, no effect comparable to estrogen has been demonstrated, but there is some preliminary evidence of the bone-preserving potential of Kampo therapy. For example, a randomized control trial in 30 surgically-menopausal osteopenic patients has shown that Cinnamon Twig and Poria Pills combined with a form of activated vitamin D3 led to a significant increase in cortical bone mass over a 10-month period, and is more effective than activated vitamin D3 alone or non-treatment.(16)

Bone health depends on multiple interacting parameters. Diet, activity level, other diseases, and drug use can all influence the processes of bone repair, formation, and resorption. Although the specific impact of traditional remedies on bones remains unclear, several interrelated features of Kampo medicine may be expected to contribute to the prevention and treatment of osteoporosis.

• Overall health

Kampo treatment increases resistance and the ability to recover from illness. It helps to raise the level of overall health, which affects bone health.

• Circulation

Bone formation and repair would be undermined if circulation to the bones were impaired. Many Kampo remedies improve circulation and may be expected to exert a positive effect in this regard.

• Nutritional factors

A proper diet is important in supplying the body with calcium and other nutrients necessary to bone health. However, the benefit of a sound diet cannot be realized unless there is also sound digestion and absorption. The improvement of GI function is a major benefit that can be derived from Kampo.

• Other illness

Developing osteoporosis often is not an isolated medical problem. Beginning with limitation of physical activity that contributes to further impairment of skeletal strength, concurrent chronic conditions may be related to osteoporosis in complex, poorly understood ways. The integrative approach of Kampo medicine to patient evaluation and treatment is desirable in such instances of comorbidy.

For example, worsening of diabetes is associated with increased rate of bone loss, and insulin-dependent diabetics have a higher-than-average risk of complications from osteoporosis. Eight-Ingredient Rehmannia Pills and kindred formulas not only can ameliorate osteoporosis-related low back pain, but also can contribute to the stabilization of diabetes mellitus in patients having the corresponding pattern. These formulas are also beneficial in atrophic vaginitis and urinary disorders.

• Drugs

A number of drugs create a negative calcium balance. For example, anti-inflammatory analgesics may cause digestive disturbances and interfere with the absorption of calcium and other nutrients. Many common antacids contain aluminum, which augments calcium loss from the body. Common anticonvulsants may interfere with vitamin D metabolism, causing decreased calcium absorption. Older people, the age group at risk for osteoporosis, tend to use more medications and thus are also at greater risk for intensifying the problem.

Steroid drugs used to control such diseases as asthma and connective tissue diseases are the most insidious offenders. Prolonged use of high doses of steroids accelerates bone loss and diminishes bone formation, and can cause depression that saps energy and reduces physical activity. Induction of severe osteoporosis is not uncommon among chronic users.(17)

Kampo may be prescribed in many instances where such drugs are being used to enable dosage reduction and possibly withdrawal. Again, this contributes indirectly to the prevention of osteoporosis.

Like estrogen therapy, the benefits of Kampo can be better realized if treatment is initiated before osteoprosis becomes established. Indeed, a judicious application of Kampo would be in the reduction of clinically modifiable risk factors in younger women at risk for osteoporosis.

A. Remedies

As may be inferred from the above discussion, numerous remedies can potentially contribute to the prevention and treatment of osteoporosis. Since they cannot all be cited here, this guideline focuses on four related therapeutic objectives:

1. Ramifications of diminished ovarian function

In perimenopausal women or younger women with ovarian underactivity (hypoestrogenic amenorrhea), the most frequently applicable formulas are Tangkuei and Peony Powder, Channel-Warming Decoction, and Cinnamon Twig and Poria Pills. Other formulas in the Hot Flushes table may also be useful.

Eight-Ingredient Rehmannia Pills and its derivatives are generally suitablein older patient populations. These are remedies traditionally employed to supplement the "kidney," which in Kampo refers to a sphere of function representing parts of the the urinary, reproductive, and endocrine systems and a part of the brain function. A role for kidney-supplementing remedies in osteoporosis is inherent in the traditional medical theory, which ascribes the growth and healing of the bones to the kidney function and associates depletion of the kidney with degenerative changes.

2. Symptomatic osteoporosis

Low back pain, and pain and sensory disturbances in the extremities are the most common symptoms related to osteoporosis. As is true for musculoskeletal problems in general, features of fluid imbalance and blood stasis are regularly observed in osteoporotic patients. Recall that both have to do with abnormal flow or distribution; in other words, impaired circulation and cellular exchange. Remedies that are likely to be useful here are basically the ones used for body aches and pains. In addition to the ones listed in the accompanying table, other formulas introduced in the preceding chapter may be considered.

3. The GI function and calcium absorption

Many formulas can be useful in normalizing the GI function and enhancing calcium absorption. In addition to the ones indicated in the table, the following may be relevant:

- Bupleurum and Cinnamon Twig Decoction
- Bupleurum, Cinnamon Twig and Dried Ginger Decoction
- Cinnamon Twig and Ginseng Decoction
- Pinellia, Ovate Atractylodes and Gastrodia Decoction
- Spleen-Returning Decoction
- True Warrior Decoction

4. General vitality

Center-Supplementing Qi-Boosting Decoction and Perfect Major Supplementation Decoction are examples of remedies that raise general vitality levels. Where indications exist, they may be employed in combination with other formulas. Furthermore, beginning with formulas suitable for weak digestive function, many Kampo formulas introduced in this manual incorporate "superior" substances (see p. 24) and have varying degress of health-building effects.

As always, formulation of the treatment plan should be guided by the overall condition of the patient. Other chapters in Part III may be consulted as needed.

B. Combination with conventional medications

The constitutional effects of Kampo treatment complement the biomedical focus on target organs. Combinations with calcium supplements, estrogen, calcitonin, etc. are possible and indeed desirable in certain cases.

C. Evaluation

Kampo treatment may be expected to ameliorate painful symptoms related to osteoporosis within two to four weeks. Long-term treatment is generally indicated to bring about constitutional improvement. Depending on the patient's subjective response and changes in bone mass status, different combinations of Kampo remedies and conventional therapies may need to be tried during the course of treatment.

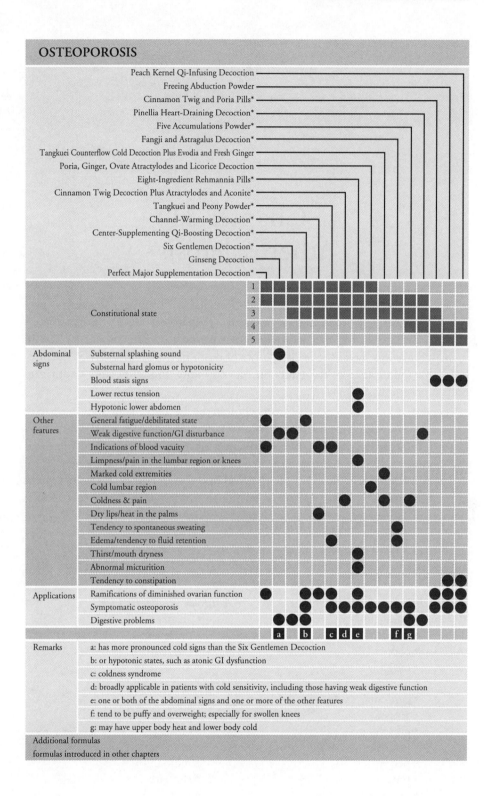

OSTEOPOROSIS

Peach Kernel Qi-Infusing Decoction
Freeing Abduction Powder
Cinnamon Twig and Poria Pills*
Pinellia Heart-Draining Decoction*
Five Accumulations Powder*
Fangji and Astragalus Decoction*
Tangkuei Counterflow Cold Decoction Plus Evodia and Fresh Ginger
Poria, Ginger, Ovate Atractylodes and Licorice Decoction
Eight-Ingredient Rehmannia Pills*
Cinnamon Twig Decoction Plus Atractylodes and Aconite*
Tangkuei and Peony Powder*
Channel-Warming Decoction*
Center-Supplementing Qi-Boosting Decoction*
Six Gentlemen Decoction*
Ginseng Decoction
Perfect Major Supplementation Decoction*

Constitutional state — 1, 2, 3, 4, 5

Abdominal signs	Substernal splashing sound
	Substernal hard glomus or hypotonicity
	Blood stasis signs
	Lower rectus tension
	Hypotonic lower abdomen
Other features	General fatigue/debilitated state
	Weak digestive function/GI disturbance
	Indications of blood vacuity
	Limpness/pain in the lumbar region or knees
	Marked cold extremities
	Cold lumbar region
	Coldness & pain
	Dry lips/heat in the palms
	Tendency to spontaneous sweating
	Edema/tendency to fluid retention
	Thirst/mouth dryness
	Abnormal micturition
	Tendency to constipation
Applications	Ramifications of diminished ovarian function
	Symptomatic osteoporosis
	Digestive problems

a b c d e f g

Remarks	
a:	has more pronounced cold signs than the Six Gentlemen Decoction
b:	or hypotonic states, such as atonic GI dysfunction
c:	coldness syndrome
d:	broadly applicable in patients with cold sensitivity, including those having weak digestive function
e:	one or both of the abdominal signs and one or more of the other features
f:	tend to be puffy and overweight; especially for swollen knees
g:	may have upper body heat and lower body cold

Additional formulas

formulas introduced in other chapters

Chapter 21
Atherosclerosis

Atherosclerotic cardiovascular disease has a lower incidence in pre-menopausal women than men in age-matched groups, but starts to increase during the perimenopausal period to a rate similar to that in men.(4) Since it is by far the leading cause of death in women in the US, the public health significance of its reduction on morbidity, mortality, and health care costs is enormous.(3)

Hypertension and elevated serum cholesterol are two major long-term risk factors for atherosclerosis which can be affected by pharmacotherapy. Like osteoporosis, they can be progressive consequences of metabolic changes initiated in the climacteric. Many Kampo remedies employed for symptomatic menopause appear to exert a favorable effect on lipid and lipoprotein metabolism and/or benefit hypertension. They may prove to be effective prophylaxis for atherosclerosis.

Pharmacology (18)

Recent animal experiments showed that many substances used in Kampo have antihypertensive and/or antihyperlipidemic effects. As examples, we cite those which are components of remedies introduced in this book:

Antihypertensive	*Antihyperlipidemic*
• astragalus	• alisma
• cinnamon	• astragalus
• coptis	• bupleurum
• fangji	• dioscorea
• uncaria	• coix
• gardenia	• coptis
• ginger	• gardenia
• ginseng	• ginseng
• jujube	• pinellia
• peony	• rehmannia
• pueraria	• rhubarb
• tangkuei	• scutellaria

Ginseng and bupleurm especially have been investigated in depth, and were shown to prevent atherosclerosis as well.

Animal data and preliminary clinical studies also suggested that Coptis Toxin-Resolving Decoction, Uncaria Powder, Major Bupleurum Decoction, and Cinnamon Twig and Poria Pills lower high blood pressure; and that the following remedies improve hyperlipidemia:

- Major Bupleurum Decoction
- Bupleurum Decoction Plus Dragon Bone and Oyster Shell
- Coptis Toxin-Resolving Decoction
- Three Yellows Heart-Draining Decoction
- Cinnamon Twig and Poria Pills
- Eight-Ingredient Rehmannia Pills
- Ledebouriella Sage-Inspired Powder

Additionally, the following substances have been shown to inhibit platelet aggregation and/or promote fibrinolysis, actions that help to halt the progression of atherosclerosis:

- bupleurum
- cinnamon
- coptis
- ginseng
- moutan
- peach kernel
- scutellaria
- tangkuei
- peony
- rhubarb

The above data suggest a pharmacological basis for the benefits of Kampo remedies. They offer some tantalizing evidence that the prevention of cardiovascular morbidity and mortality, a major long-range goal of HRT, can also be promoted with Kampo. Needless to say, further research is required to elucidate the possible mechanisms of actions and to provide conclusive demonstration of the value of Kampo therapy in cardiovascular risk reduction.

Kampo treatment

Hyperlipidemia

Kampo examination does not identify high serum cholesterol levels per se, nor does Kampo treatment aim specifically at the improvement of the lipid profile. However, people with diagnosed hyperlipidemia often exhibit signs of caloric excess, constipation, and signs of blood stasis.[1] Kampo treatment aims to ameliorate these and other signs and symptoms of imbalance, and can bring about desirable modifications of lipid levels in the process.

---

[1] *From a modern perspective, the increase in blood viscosity and tendency to form clots seen in hyperlipidemia suggests a role for Kampo blood stasis remedies.*

In general, Kampo therapy is more effective than diet management in lowering elevated blood lipids, but not as effective as modern hypolipidemic drugs. It is therefore suitable for relatively mild cases which comprise the majority. It could be especially useful for the elderly, in whom drug side effects are an important concern and diet management may seriously impair the quality of life through the restriction of favored foods. Where drugs are indicated, Kampo can also be employed as an adjunct to improve overall condition.

Hypertension

As in hyperlipidemia, Kampo treatment aims to alleviate subjective symptoms and to improve overall health. This complements the Western treatment objective of blood pressure reduction.

The subjective symptoms accompanying hypertension respond well to Kampo. They commonly include headrushes, hyperemia of eye membranes, irritability, nervousness, anxiety, palpitations, insomnia, headache, heavy-headedness, stiff shoulders, tinnitus, urinary frequency, and coldness conditions.

Blood pressure may decrease gradually as a consequence of Kampo therapy, but in many cases it does not. Antihypertensive drugs are superior in simply lowering the blood pressure. Kampo is most valuble in the management of mild labile or borderline cases of essential hypertension, where the risks of drug therapy generally outweigh its benefits; and in cases with many psychosomatic symptoms. The gradual, progressive action of Kampo remedies can be particularly suitable in the elderly, in whom too quick or too much pressure reduction can easily provoke postural hypotension and other complications.

A. Remedies

The clinical manifestations of both hypertension and hyperlipidemia are similar. The same group of remedies can be applied.

B. Evaluation

Improvement in subjective symptoms should be observed within two to three weeks of therapy. Stabilization of blood pressure follows, but a significant reduction is not always observed. For borderline to mild cases of high serum cholesterol (approx. 220-300 mg/dl), a 10-20% reduction is possible following three months of treatment.

C. Combination with conventional medication

In more serious cases of hypertension or hyperlipidemia, Kampo may be employed adjunctively to treat subjective symptoms not alleviated by drugs and possibly enable a gradual reduction of drug dosage. Kampo therapy can also prevent or ameliorate drug side effects, such as the increase of serum uric acid or increase in blood sugar level associated with diuretic drugs, liver function impairment associated with ACE inhibitors, elevation of serum lipids associated with beta blockers, or gastrointestinal side effects associated with bile-acids absorbing resins.

Antihypertensive drugs work by many different mechanisms. It remains to be determined which types are most suitable to combine with Kampo. Currently, ACE inhibitors and calcium channel blockers appear to be favored by Japanese physicians.

D. Caution

Reduction of antihypertensive drugs (notably those with central sympatholytic action) should be gradual, as abrupt withdrawal can have serious rebound effects.

The risk of combining a potassium-wasting diuretic agent with licorice-containing Kampo formulas has been mentioned elsewhere in this manual. Undesirable pharmacokinetic interactions are also possible between certain Kampo remedies and hypolipidemic drugs. Kampo remedies that inhibit the absorption of dietary lipids can lower the uptake of a highly lipid-soluble drug such as Clofibrate®. Resins, on the other hand, can interfere with the absorption of Kampo remedies.

Self-help measures

• Commonsense measures such as dietary modifications, weight reduction, and exercise should be undertaken.

• Meditation and relaxation techniques can help to alleviate stress contributing to hypertension.

HYPERTENSION • HYPERLIPIDEMIA

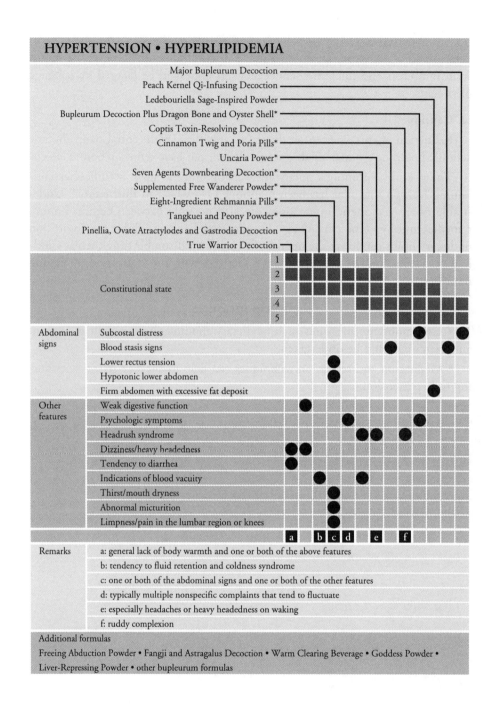

Major Bupleurum Decoction
Peach Kernel Qi-Infusing Decoction
Ledebouriella Sage-Inspired Powder
Bupleurum Decoction Plus Dragon Bone and Oyster Shell*
Coptis Toxin-Resolving Decoction
Cinnamon Twig and Poria Pills*
Uncaria Power*
Seven Agents Downbearing Decoction*
Supplemented Free Wanderer Powder*
Eight-Ingredient Rehmannia Pills*
Tangkuei and Peony Powder*
Pinellia, Ovate Atractylodes and Gastrodia Decoction
True Warrior Decoction

Constitutional state
1
2
3
4
5

Abdominal signs
Subcostal distress
Blood stasis signs
Lower rectus tension
Hypotonic lower abdomen
Firm abdomen with excessive fat deposit

Other features
Weak digestive function
Psychologic symptoms
Headrush syndrome
Dizziness/heavy headedness
Tendency to diarrhea
Indications of blood vacuity
Thirst/mouth dryness
Abnormal micturition
Limpness/pain in the lumbar region or knees

a b c d e f

Remarks
a: general lack of body warmth and one or both of the above features
b: tendency to fluid retention and coldness syndrome
c: one or both of the abdominal signs and one or both of the other features
d: typically multiple nonspecific complaints that tend to fluctuate
e: especially headaches or heavy headedness on waking
f: ruddy complexion

Additional formulas

Freeing Abduction Powder • Fangji and Astragalus Decoction • Warm Clearing Beverage • Goddess Powder • Liver-Repressing Powder • other bupleurum formulas

References for Part III

(1) Notelovitz, Morris. "Estrogen Replacement Therapy: Indications, Contraindications and Agent Selection." *American Journal of Obstetrics and Gynecology* 161 (1989): 1832-41.

(2) Kase, Nathan G. "The management of the postmenopausal woman." In *Postmenopausal Hormonal Therapy: Benefits and Risks,* edited by Piero Fioretti *et al.* New York: Raven Press, 1987, pp.35-54.

(3) Booher, Delbert L. "Estrogen Supplements in Menopause." *Cleveland Clinic Journal of Medicine 57* (1990): 154-160.

(4) Utian, Wulf H. "Biosynthesis and Physiologic Effects of Estrogen and Pathophysiologic Effects of Estrogen Deficiency: A Review." *American Journal of Obstetrics and Gynecology 161* (1989): 1828-31.

(5) Nachtigall, Lila and Joan Rattner Heilman. *Estrogen: The Facts Can Change Your Life.* New York: Harper and Row, 1986, pp.61-63.

(6) Hunter, Myra S. "Emotional Well-Being, Sexual Behaviour and Hormone Replacement Therapy." *Maturitas* 12 (1990): 299-314.

(7) Fink, Paul J. "Psychiatric Myths of the Menopause." In *The Menopause: Comprehensive Management,* edited by Bernard Eskin. New York: MacMillan, 1988.

(8a) London, Steve and Jane Chihal. *Menopause: Clinical Concepts.* Essential Medical Information Systems, Inc., 1989, p. 93.

(8b) *Ibid.,* p. 114.

(8c) *Ibid.,* p. 88-89.

(8d) *Ibid.,* p. 78-79.

(9) Narita, Hiro-o. "Kōutsuzai Fukusayō Kanwa" (Alleviation of Side Effects of Antidepressive Medications). No. 72 of The Latest Kampo Treatment Guidelines, *Journal of Japanese Medical Association,* June 15, 1986.

(10) Aono, Toshihiro. "Hairan Shōgai" (Ovulatory Dysfunction). *Journal of Japanese Medical Association* 106:8 (1991): RK77-80.

(11) Barber, Hugh R.K. "Gynecologic Problems." In *The Menopause: Comprehensive Management,* edited by Bernard Eskin. New York: MacMillan, 1988.

(12) Dalton, Katharina. *The Premenstrual Syndrome and Progesterone Therapy* (2nd edition). London: William Heinemann Medical Books Ltd., 1984, pp. 215-224.

(13a) Sutherst J.R. *et al. Introduction to Clinical Gynaecological Urology.* London: Butterworth-Heinemann Ltd., 1990, Chapter 11.

(13b) *Ibid.,* Chapters 4 & 9.

(14) Karafin, Lester. "Urologic Problems." In *The Menopause: Comprehensive Management,* edited by Bernard Eskin. New York: MacMillan, 1988.

(15) Mellstrom D. *et al.* "Special health services: An introduction to a programme for elderly women with urinary incontinence and related symptoms." *Maturitas* 9 (1988):289-296.

(16) Ōta, Hiroaki. "Ransō Zentekigo Kotsuenryō Genshō Shō" ("Osteopenia Following Oophorectomy"). *Journal of the Japanese Medical Association* 101:8 (1989):KS1-2.

(17) Fardon, David F. "Osteoporosis: Your head start on the prevention & treatment of brittle bones." *The Body Press,* pp. 60-63.

(18) Matsuda, Kunio and Kazumoto Inaki. *Rinshōi no Tame no Kampō (Kampo for Clinicians).* Current Therapy Inc., 1987, pp. 136-7, 171-2.

PART IV
FORMULAS AND PATTERNS

Preliminary Considerations

Numerous versions of formula patterns are found in contemporary Kampo literature. Collectively, they are products of exegeses by latter generations of clinicians upon the classical descriptions of the patterns. Depending on the orientation and sophistication of the intended audience, they range from simple lists of clinical features to monographs including discussions of the pathologies treated by the formula, the properties of its component substances, and differential diagnosis.

The representation in this book is one in a series of attempts to render the application of Kampo formulas more intelligible to modern users. It differentiates itself in being specifically adapted for use by practitioners in the West within the context of climacteric symptomatology.

Format

The entries are arranged alphabetically by the English names of the formula. Each entry comprises the following parts:

1. Names
- English name of the formula
- Japanese name
- Chinese Pinyin name

2. Composition
Component substances and their daily dosages in grams.[1]

3. Pattern
Features of the pattern are grouped under the following headings:

---

[1] *With few exceptions, the composition is as specified in the Handbook of General-Use Kampo Formulas (Ippanyō Kampō Shohō no Tebiki) edited by the Pharmaceutical Affairs Bureau of the Japanese Ministry of Health and Welfare, and reflects the possible variation of component dosages in Japanese commercial extract preparations. The composition of formulas not included in the Handbook derives from classical sources. Note that doasages in Kampo are generally about 1/3 of dosages current in Chinese medicine.*

This information does not reflect the substitution of constituents that can occur in practice. For instance, cinnamon bark is employed in place of cinnamon twig in Japanese extract preparations, and fresh ginger, dried ginger, and dried steamed ginger are often used interchangeably. Such distinctions are beyond the scope of this book.

- **Constitutional state**

A composite index of abdominal strength and other findings pertaining to reserve and resistance (see p. 36). Rated by a five-level scale: five represents sthenia, one represents asthenia. Parentheses indicate the applicable range.

- **Typical traits/predisposing factors**

Somatic and psychological tendencies, lifestyle factors, and other factors contributing to the condition of imbalance. Cited if the association is generally acknowledged. This information helps to identify the typical patient type.

- **Signs and symptoms**

The major and minor signs and symptoms, including abdominal findings where relevant. Please see Chapter 5, p. 34, "Content of a pattern" for an explanation of major and minor features, and Chapter 8, p. 75, for the diagnostic criteria recommended in this manual.

Efforts have been made to avoid unwieldy lists. In place of the straightforward enumeration of features found in many introductory-level Japanese texts, signs and symptoms are categorized as much as is possible by the basic concepts of pathology discussed in Chapter 5: asthenia and sthenia, cold and heat, coldness syndrome, headrush syndrome, blood imbalances (blood stasis, blood vacuity), fluid imbalances, and weak digestive function. Apart from gains in organization, this approach has the advantage of helping the user to develop a better grasp of the nature of the condition treated with a particular formula.

Asthenia or sthenia forms a category in addition to the five-level scale above when certain aspects of the constitutional state are important in pattern delineation. Weak digestive function, though a subset of asthenia, can also be a major heading when the pattern warrants the emphasis. Headrush or headrush syndrome is usually subsumed under the categories of "heat," "cold/heat" or "others," depending on the other items present.

Familiar English terms such as "GI disturbances" and "Psychologic symptoms" are also used as headings if they adequately summarize a group of signs and symptoms. "Others" is a catch-all category for lone items, or miscellaneous items that are difficult to classify on the basis of the general pathological concepts introduced in this book.

Some items potentially fit multiple categories since the latter are interrelated and overlap to various extents. In such cases, assignments of the items were based on personal judgement.

Underlines indicate major features. If a category is underlined, it means one or more of the items it contains have principal significance. Unless indicated otherwise, items listed on separate lines under a category always stand in an "and/or" relationship with each other; that is, one or more items may apply. Multiple items in the same line separated by comma(s) without further qualifications are to be interpreted likewise. The latter is typically done for reasons of spatial economy and ease of reading in the case of items that tend to be alternatives or to occur in tandem, or items that express different intensity of the phenomenon in question. Examples are "headaches, heavy-headedness," "nausea, vomiting," and diverse items under the category of Psychologic symptoms.

Finally, the list given is not exhaustive. Uncommon findings have been excluded. With the exception of some formulas for joint and muscle pains, the signs and symptoms listed are primarily those relevant to chronic disorders. Many formulas were used in the past in febrile diseases, so fever, etc., may indeed be part of the pattern. This may be inferred from the "Additional Applications" section.

• TCM pattern identification

This information is provided for users familiar with the patterns of disharmony identified in Traditional Chinese Medicine.

4. Applications

Conditions discussed in Part III in which the formula may be beneficial.

5. Additional applications

Representative disorders in which the pattern may be identified. Intended to impart a feel for the potential range of applications of a formula.

6. Notes

This section includes notes on differential diagnosis, points on administration, precautions, additions, combinations, etc., which are useful in clinical practice.

Component substances on the Caution List (Appendix A) are also enumerated here. In particular, common formula ingredients whose misuse is more likely to engender problems are flagged by an asterisk: aconite, ephedra, mirabilite, rehmannia, rhubarb, and licorice if the daily dose exceeds 2.5g.[2] Note that this is a mechanical listing of all ingredients on the Caution List. Depending on the dose of the substance in question and the overall composition, the potential for adverse effects associated with prudent application of the formula may be negligible. Nevertheless, to ensure the safety of treatment, the practitioner should always take careful notice of this information when making therapeutic decisions.

Personal Insight

Any verbal rendition of a pattern, however replete with detail, is no more than a general guideline on the application of a formula. Ultimately, each practitioner must map the terrain of utility on his or her own. There is no substitute to the accumulation of clinical experience in comprehending a formula's utmost scope of efficacy.

---

[2] *See Section V of Appendix A for precautions regarding pregnancy.*

BUPLEURUM AND CINNAMON TWIG DECOCTION
Saikokeishitō   *chái hú guì zhī tāng*

COMPOSITION

bupleurum	5g.	peony	2-3g.	jujube	2g.
pinellia	4g.	scutellaria	2g.	licorice	1.5-2g.
cinnamon twig	2-3g.	ginseng	2g.	dried ginger	1g.

PATTERN

Constitutional state   5 (4 3 2) 1

Signs and symptoms

Psychologic symptoms .... • tension, irritability, depressed mood, insomnia

GI disturbances .... • substernal discomfort or pain

            • nausea, vomiting

            • loss of appetite

Others .... • tendency toward headrushes, headaches, or spontaneous sweating

            • neck and shoulder stiffness

Abdominal findings .... • mild subcostal distress

            • upper rectus tension (and possibly tenderness) and/or substernal hard glomus

TCM pattern identification

Binding depression of liver qi or liver-stomach disharmony, with signs of spleen qi vacuity and phlegm-damp

APPLICATIONS

Hot flushes and other vasomotor manifestations

Sleep disturbances............... • can be effective for difficulty in maintaining sleep or nonrestorative sleep

Emotional distress.............. • neurotic conditions (including gastrointestinal neurosis), nervous exhaustion, premenstrual tension, etc.

Chronic headaches.............. • tension headaches, migraines

Body aches and pains.......... • may be beneficial for stiffness and pain in the neck and shoulder area

Hypertension, hyperlipidemia, atherosclerosis ....

            • can be useful in cases where stress appears to be a significant etiologic factor

ADDITIONAL APPLICATIONS

Digestive .... • gastritis, gastric hyperacidity, peptic ulcer, inflammatory bowel disease, irritable bowel syndrome, pancreatitis, hepatitis, gallstones

Gynecologic .... • PMS, psychogenic amenorrhea, adnexitis

EENT .... • myopia spuria, sinusitis, allergic rhinitis, recurrent otitis media

Skin .... • urticaria, chloasma, excessive hair loss

Others .... • febrile diseases (common cold, influenza, bronchitis, etc.), peritonitis, nephrosis, neuralgia, epilepsy

NOTES

May be applied as a constitutional alterative in individuals having a tendency to suffer from allergy-based disorders or to contract colds easily.

Substances on the Caution List: cinnamon, ginger, ginseng, jujube, licorice, peony, pinellia.

BUPLEURUM, CINNAMON TWIG AND DRIED GINGER DECOCTION
Saikokeishikankyōtō   *chái hú guì jiāng tāng*

COMPOSITION

bupleurum	5-6g.	scutellaria	3g.	licorice	2g.
cinnamon twig	3g.	oyster shell	3g.		
trichosanthes root	3-4g.	dried ginger	2g.		

PATTERN

Constitutional state   5 4 (3 2 1)

Typical traits/predisposing factors
Fatigue, easy fatigability
Thin physique, pallor

Signs and symptoms

Fluid imbalance .... • thirst, or mild mouth and throat dryness
 • spontaneous sweating (or night sweating) from the head
 • reduced urinary output

Psychologic symptoms .... • restlessness, marked sense of fatigue, irritability, anxiety, overreaction to stimuli (increased startle response), depressed mood, insomnia, etc.

Cold/Heat .... • cold extremities (possibly also coldness in the back)
 • headrush syndrome–associated symptoms include sweating from the head, headaches, or heavy-headedness

Others .... • palpitations
 • neck and shoulder stiffness

Abdominal findings .... • periumbilical pulsation (possibly with subjective awareness of the pulsation)
 • slight subcostal distress
 • tender point immediately inferior to the xiphoid process and tenderness over the sternum

TCM pattern identification
Binding depression of liver qi and disquieted spirit, with vacuity of liquid and cold signs

APPLICATIONS

Hot flushes and other vasomotor manifestations
Sleep disturbances .... • difficulty in initiating or maintaining sleep, nonrestorative sleep, dream-troubled sleep

- Emotional distress .... • anxiety, depression, nervous exhaustion, neurotic conditions
- Chronic headaches .... • applicable in migraines, tension headaches, mixed headaches, etc.
- Body aches and pains ...... • may be beneficial for stiffness and pain in the neck and shoulder area

ADDITIONAL APPLICATIONS

Digestive .... • hyperacidity, gastric ulcer, chronic hepatitis, jaundice

EENT .... • myopia spuria, recurrent otitis media, allergic rhinitis

Skin .... • chloasma, urticaria, excessive hair loss

Hormonal-metabolic .... • hyperthyroidism, diabetes

Others .... • febrile disorders (common cold, influenza, bronchitis, pneumonia, pulmonary tuberculosis), nephrosis

NOTES

This formula may be considered the asthenic counterpart of Bupleurum Decoction Plus Dragon Bone and Oyster Shell in the above five applications.

In the past, it was frequently applied in pulmonary tuberculosis and malaria-like diseases. Nowadays it is most often prescribed in psychosomatic disorders and neurotic conditions.

Substances on the Caution List: cinnamon, ginger, licorice.

BUPLEURUM DECOCTION PLUS DRAGON BONE AND OYSTER SHELL
Saikokaryūkotsuboreitō   chái hú jiā lóng gǔ mǔ lì tāng

COMPOSITION

bupleurum	4-5g.	jujube	2-2.5g.	fresh ginger	2-3g.
pinellia	4g.	ginseng	2-2.5g.	scutellaria	0-2.5g.
poria	2-3g.	dragon bone	2-2.5g.	rhubarb	0-1g.
cinnamon twig	2-3g.	oyster shell	2-2.5g.		

(May be formulated with or without rhubarb, scutellaria, and licorice. Up to 2g. of licorice may be incorporated in some preparations.)

PATTERN

Constitutional state: (5 4 3) 2 1

Signs and symptoms

Psychologic symptoms .... • restlessness, overreaction to stimuli (increased startle response), anxiety, irritability, mood swings, depressed mood, introversion, sense of fatigue, difficulty concentrating, insomnia, etc.

Fluid imbalance .... • sense of heaviness/cumbersomeness

• edema

• reduced urinary output

Others .... • palpitations (often triggered by a startle reaction)

• headrush syndrome–associated symptoms include heavy-headedness, headaches, dizziness, tinnitus

• neck and shoulder stiffness

Abdominal findings .... • subcostal distress

• periumbilical pulsation (possibly with subjective awareness of the pulsation)

• substernal hard glomus

TCM pattern identification

Disquieted spirit and depressed heat of liver and gallbladder, with signs of spleen qi vacuity and phlegm-damp

APPLICATIONS

Hot flushes and other vasomotor manifestations

Sleep disturbances .... • difficulty in initiating or maintaining sleep, nonrestorative sleep, dream-troubled sleep, excessive sleepiness, etc.

> • may possibly induce vivid dreams in persons who do not usually remember dreaming

Emotional distress .... • anxiety, depression, neurotic conditions

> • the cumbersomeness often present in depressive states may be due in part to fluid retention. This formula will lighten the body by ridding it of excess fluid

Chronic headaches

Urinary disorders .... • may be beneficial for urethral syndrome or other urinary dysfunctions with the above pattern

Body aches and pains .... • may be beneficial for stiffness and pain in the neck and shoulder area

Hypertension, hyperlipidemia, atherosclerosis ....

> • suitable for psychosomatic cardiovascular disease

> • commonly employed in contemporary Japan alongside antihypertensive drugs as an alternative to biomedical minor tranquilizers

> • can be applied in long-term treatment of angina and cerebrovascular disorders

ADDITIONAL APPLICATIONS

Hyperthyroidism, epilepsy, stroke aftereffects (hemiplegia), nephrosis, nephritis, excessive hair loss, psychosis

NOTES

Sthenic-appearing individuals weakened by illness may on occasion experience a worsening of palpitations and anxiety with the use of this formula. Switch to a more asthenic-oriented formula if this occurs.

A small amount of Coptis Toxin-Resolving Decoction may be added in cases with marked irritability and other heat symptoms.

The inclusion of scutellaria (omitted in some preparations) is desirable.

The rhubarb-less version is suitable if abdominal pain or diarrhea results from taking the rhubarb-containing version.

Substances on the Caution List: cinnamon, ginger, ginseng, jujube, pinellia; (*rhubarb, licorice).

CENTER-SUPPLEMENTING QI-BOOSTING DECOCTION
Hochūekkitō   *bǔ zhōng yì qì tāng*

COMPOSITION

ginseng	4g.	tangerine peel	2g.	dried ginger	0.5g.
ovate atractylodes	4g.	jujube	2g.	cimicifuga	0.5-1g.
astragalus	3-4g.	bupleurum	1-2g.		
tangkuei	3g.	licorice	1-1.5g.		

PATTERN

Constitutional state   5 4 (3 2 1)

Signs and symptoms

<u>Generalized chronic or acute fatigue, lack of energy, adynamia; or fatigue/hypotonic state of muscles and support tissues</u> (prolapse of internal organs, lowered tonus of the digestive tract, poor sphincter tone, etc.), typically with one or more of the following manifestations:

Asthenia .... • languid extremities
• inability to maintain a gaze (lack of force in
• the eyes/dull eyes)
• lethargy after eating
• spontaneous sweating, night sweating
• voice without energy

Depressed digestive function... • poor appetite
• preference for warm food and drink
• insensitivity to taste
• bloating

Others .... • low grade fever or feverish feeling
• accompanying fatigue

Abdominal findings .... • periumbilical pulsation
• slight subcostal distress
• sagging of the abdomen

TCM pattern identification

Qi vacuity, spleen-stomach qi vacuity, center qi fall, spleen failing to manage the blood (qi failing to contain the blood), defense qi vacuity

APPLICATIONS

Abnormal bleeding/menstrual disorders/vaginal symptoms ....
• may be beneficial for prolapse of the uterus or
chronic abnormal uterine bleeding (chronic
intermittent loss of small amounts of blood)

Urinary disorders .... • may be beneficial in incontinence and other
urinary problems associated with insufficient
bladder and sphincter tone, or pelvic relaxation

Body aches and pains, osteoporosis ....
• may be applied in chronic low back pain with
the above pattern
• may be beneficial in osteoporosis (helps restore
vitality, also suitable for atonic GI dysfunctions)

ADDITIONAL APPLICATIONS

Digestive .... • gastritis, constipation or diarrhea from
gastrointestinal atony, chronic hepatitis,
liver cirrhosis

Respiratory .... • pleurisy, tuberculosis, bronchitis, common cold

EENT .... • eye fatigue, asthenopia, amblyopia

Others .... • prolapse of internal organs, convalescence,
post-operative disorders (dumping syndrome,
fecal or urinary incontinence, etc.), low blood
pressure, hypothyroidism

NOTES

A representative remedy to restore the vitality.

May be applied as a constitutional alterative for asthenia. Improves overall energy and boosts the functioning of the immune system when taken over time. May also be employed prior to some enervating undertaking or procedure (e.g., surgery, radiation therapy) to prevent or reduce debilitation in susceptible persons.

Also suitable in ordinarily sthenic individuals for acute fatigue or loss of energy.

Beneficial as an adjunct to drug or radiation treatment that causes malaise, anemia, anorexia, GI and liver problems; and to speed recovery from surgical operations.

Perfect Major Supplementation Decoction should be considered in cases with evident blood vacuity or significant wasting of the material aspect of the body.

Substances on the Caution List: ginger, ginseng, jujube, licorice, tangkuei.

Contraindications: In general, avoid long-term use in individuals with high blood pressure because of possible hypertensive effects. Not suitable for severely debilitated conditions.

CHANNEL-COURSING BLOOD-QUICKENING DECOCTION
Sokeikakketsutō   *shū jīng huó xuè tāng*

COMPOSITION

tangkuei	2g.	peony	2.5g.	gentian	1.5g.
rehmannia	2g.	achyranthes	1.5g.	tangerine peel	1.5g.
ligusticum	2g.	clematis	1.5g.	fresh ginger	1-1.5g.
atractylodes root	2g.	fangji	1.5g.	angelica	1-1.5g.
poria	2g.	notopterygium	1.5g.	licorice	1g.
peach kernel	2g.	ledebouriella	1.5g.		

PATTERN

Constitutional state   5 (4 3 2) 1

Signs and symptoms

Chronic rheumatic afflictions.... • arthralgia, myalgia, neuralgia (pain possibly more severe at night)
• edema
• stiffness, impeded movement
• numbness

Blood imbalance .... • lusterless skin
• paresthesia
• muscle spasm

Abdominal findings .... • may have blood stasis signs

TCM pattern identification

Wind-damp bi with signs of blood vacuity and blood stasis

APPLICATIONS

Body aches and pains .... • arthritis, low back pain, sciatica, fibrositis

ADDITIONAL APPLICATIONS

Gout, beriberi, aftereffects of stroke (hemiplegia)

NOTES

This formula is most often prescribed for aches and pains in the lumbar region and below. Though traditionally reputed to be especially suitable for pain in the left lower extremity or pain that is more severe at night, it may be applied broadly in all rhumatic conditions with features of blood and fluid imbalances.

Combine with an appropriate blood stasis formula if features of blood stasis are pronounced.

Substances on the Caution List: achyranthes, ginger, ledebouriella, licorice, ligusticum, notopterygium, peach kernel, peony, *rehmannia, tangkuei.

CHANNEL-WARMING DECOCTION

Unkeitō   *wēn jīng tāng*

COMPOSITION

pinellia	3-5g.	moutan	2g.	ligusticum	2g.
tangkuei	2-3g.	dried ginger	1g.	ginseng	2g.
peony	2g.	evodia	1-3g.	ass hide glue	2g.
cinnamon twig	2g.	ophipogon	3-10g.	licorice	2g.

PATTERN

Constitutional state   5 4 (3 2 1)

Signs and symptoms

Cold/Heat............................• coldness syndrome (cold lower body and lower extremities)
• pain accompanying coldness in the lower abdomen or lumbar region
• heat in the palms (particularly at night)
• headrushes

Blood imbalance.................. • dry lips, chapped lips, dry lusterless skin, and other symptoms of blood vacuity
• menstrual disorders
• abnormal uterine bleeding

Abdominal findings.............. • generally soft; blood stasis signs possible

TCM pattern identification

Lower burner vacuity cold and blood vacuity, with signs of blood stasis and yin vacuity

APPLICATIONS

Hot flushes and other vasomotor manifestations

Abnormal bleeding/menstrual disorders/vaginal symptoms ....
• dysfunctional uterine bleeding, dysmenorrhea, irregular menstruation, PMS, abnormal vaginal discharge, atrophic vaginitis

ADDITIONAL APPLICATIONS

Gynecologic ....• amenorrhea, habitual abortion, hypoplasia uteri, infertility, endometriosis, pelvic inflammatory disease

Skin ....• hand eczema, chilblains, psoriasis

NOTES

Substances on the Caution List: cinnamon, evodia, ginger, ginseng, licorice, ligusticum, moutan, peony, pinellia, tangkuei.

CINNAMON TWIG AND GINSENG DECOCTION
Keishininjintō   *guì zhī rén shēn tāng*

COMPOSITION

cinnamon twig	4g.	ovate atractylodes	3g.	dried ginger	2g.
ginseng	3g.	licorice	3g.		

PATTERN

Constitutional state   5 4 3 (2 1)

Signs and symptoms

Weak digestive function ..... • poor appetite
• substernal discomfort
• bloating or pain
• excessive salivation or mouth dryness
• nausea, vomiting
• tendency to diarrhea (less commonly, constipation)
• sluggishness or drowsiness after eating

Coldness syndrome .... • cold sensitivity (acute GI symptoms typically precipitated by exposure to cold or excessive consumption of cold foods and drinks)
• cold extremities
• long voidings of clear urine, frequent urination

Others .... • headaches or tendency to headrushes
• tendency to spontaneous sweating

Abdominal findings .... • substernal hard glomus (or hypotonicity)
• substernal splashing sound (or less commonly, general rectus tension)

TCM pattern identification

Spleen-stomach yang vacuity (with exterior cold), or
direct strike of center by cold pathogen

APPLICATIONS

Chronic headaches .... • headaches or migraine attacks that may be accompanied by diarrhea or nausea and vomiting

ADDITIONAL APPLICATIONS

GI .... • chronic diarrhea, irritable bowel syndrome, gastroenteritis, gastric atony

Others .... • common cold, influenza

NOTE

Substances on the Caution List: cinnamon, ginger, ginseng, *licorice.

CINNAMON TWIG AND PORIA PILLS

Keishibukuryōgan   *guì zhī fú líng wán*

COMPOSITION

cinnamon twig	4g.	moutan	4g.	peony	4g.
poria	4g.	peach kernel	4g.		

PATTERN

Constitutional state   (5 4 3) 2 1

Signs and symptoms

Blood stasis ....
- indications of blood stasis in the pelvic area – menstrual disorders, abnormal genital bleeding, pelvic congestion syndrome, etc.
- other local or general indications of blood stasis

Cold/Heat ....
- headrush syndrome – associated symptoms include headrushes, neck and shoulder stiffness, headaches, dizziness, palpitations, tinnitus
- cold extremities or lower body (or upper body heat and lower body cold)

Abdominal findings ....
- blood stasis signs

TCM pattern identification

Blood stasis

APPLICATIONS

Hot flushes and other vasomotor manifestations

Emotional distress ....
- mild emotional symptoms associated with menstrual disorders and other blood stasis conditions

Chronic headaches

Abnormal bleeding/menstrual disorders/vaginal symptoms ....
- dysfunctional uterine bleeding, dysmenorrhea, irregular menstruation, PMS, atrophic vaginitis, vaginitis

Urinary disorders ....
- may be useful in conditions with blood stasis

Body aches and pains, osteoporosis ....
- low back pain, sciatica, fibrositis
- may be beneficial in osteoporosis

Hypertension, hyperlipidemia, atherosclerosis ....
- may also be beneficial in the prevention and treatment of stroke

| **ADDITIONAL APPLICATIONS** |
| Gynecologic .... • fibroids, pelvic inflammatory disease, endometriosis, infertility, habitual abortion, retention of placenta |
| Skin .... • urticaria, acne, chilblains, dermatitis, chloasma, hand eczema, psoriasis, purpura, pattern baldness |
| Eye .... • blepharitis, iritis, sty |
| CV .... • varicose veins, hemorrhoids |
| Others .... • chronic headaches, injuries, disorders associated with blood stasis |

| **NOTES** |

This is a basic formula for blood stasis conditions. It finds wide use as an adjunct to other Kampo remedies or Western drugs in disorders with features of blood stasis.

See Notes under Peach Kernel Qi-Infusing Decoction.

Add rhubarb (as needed) and licorice (extract equivalent of 1.0-2.0 g/day) in cases with constipation. Or consider Peach Kernel Qi-Infusing Decoction.

Substances on the Caution List: cinnamon, moutan, peach kernel, peony.

CINNAMON TWIG DECOCTION PLUS ATRACTYLODES AND ACONITE
Keishikajutsubutō   *guì zhī jiā zhú fù tāng*

COMPOSITION

cinnamon twig	4g.	fresh ginger	4g.	processed aconite	0.5-1g.
peony	4g.	licorice	2g.		
jujube	4g.	ovate atractylodes	4g.		

PATTERN

Constitutional state   5 4 (3 2 1)

Signs and symptoms

Rheumatic afflictions .... • arthralgia, myalgia, neuralgia
• numbness
• stiffness, impeded movement
• local swelling

Cold .... • coldness in the affected area
• symptoms worsened by cold and alleviated by warmth
• coldness syndrome

Others .... • tendency to headrushes
• tendency to spontaneous sweating
• reduced urinary output (or possibly frequency)

TCM pattern identification
cold bi

APPLICATIONS

Body aches and pains .... • arthritis, low back pain, sciatica, fibrositis

ADDITIONAL APPLICATIONS

Stroke (hemiplegia), pain from old injuries, common cold, influenza, neuropathy associated with diabetes

NOTES

Broadly applicable in asthenic patients with cold sensitivity, including those having weak digestive function.

Prescribe Cinnamon Twig Decoction Plus Poria, Atractylodes and Aconite in cases with more pronounced fluid stagnation (e.g., edema and decreased urinary output, substernal splashing sound).

Substances on the Caution List: *aconite, cinnamon, ginger, jujube, licorice, peony.

Contraindication: This formula has a strong diuretic action. Do not use if there is depletion of body fluids.

CINNAMON TWIG DECOCTION PLUS DRAGON BONE AND OYSTER SHELL
Keishikaryūkotsuboreitō　　*guì zhī jiā lóng gǔ mǔ lì tāng*

COMPOSITION

cinnamon twig	3-4g.	fresh ginger	3-4g.	oyster shell	3g.
peony	3-4g.	licorice root	2g.		
jujube	3-4g.	dragon bone	2-3g.		

PATTERN

Constitutional state　　5 4 3 (2 1)

Typical traits/predisposing factors

thin physique, pallor

Signs and symptoms

Asthenia .... • easy fatigability, fatigue
cold extremities

<u>Nervous excitability</u> .... • strongly expressed through vasomotor symptoms such as sweating, palpitations, headrushes, dizziness; with psychologic symptoms such as nervousness, anxiety, overreaction to stimuli (increased startle response), insomnia

Others .... • frequent urination
• neurotic symptoms involving genito-urinary system
• excessive hair loss

Abdominal findings .... • <u>periumbilical pulsation</u> (possibly with subjective awareness of the pulsation)
• thin wall with lower or general rectus tension

TCM pattern identification
Floating of vacuous yang, with insufficiency of qi and blood

APPLICATIONS

• Hot flushes and other vasomotor manifestations
• Sleep disturbances .... • difficulty in initiating or maintaining sleep, non-restorative sleep, dream-troubled sleep
• Emotional distress .... • nervous exhaustion, neurotic disorders involving the genito-urinary system (with symptoms such as frequent urination, dream intercourse, enuresis), other neurotic conditions
• Urinary disorders .... • urethral syndrome, nocturia, incontinence

ADDITIONAL APPLICATIONS

Arteriosclerosis, hyperthyroidism, epilepsy, nocturnal emission, and impotence in men

NOTES

Substances on the Caution List: cinnamon, ginger, jujube, licorice, peony.

COIX DECOCTION

Yokuinintō   *yì yǐ rén tāng*

COMPOSITION

ephedra	4g.	coix seed	8-10g.	licorice	2g.
tangkuei	4g.	cinnamon twig	3g.		
actractylodes	4g.	peony	3g.		

PATTERN

Constitutional state   5 (4 3) 2 1

Signs and symptoms

Chronic or subacute rheumatic afflictions ....

- arthralgia, myalgia, neuralgia with edema or sense of leaden heaviness
- local heat and rubor (mild degree, without thirst)
- stiffness, impeded movement
- numbness
- mild degree of chills or cold sensitivity

Others ....• dry skin

TCM pattern identification

Damp bi

APPLICATIONS

Body aches and pains ....• arthritis, low back pain, sciatica, fibrositis

- can be applied in cases with or without rubor and heat; pain is relatively mild and often does not improve significantly with the application of heat

ADDITIONAL APPLICATIONS

Beriberi, nephritis, tubercular arthritis

NOTES

Powdered corydalis tuber (1.0-1.5 g./day) may be added to increase the analgesic action of this formula.

See note on ephedra in Appendix A. To minimize the possibility of adverse effects from misuse of this formula, start with a small dose or have the patient take it after eating.

Substances on the Caution List: cinnamon, coix, *ephedra, licorice, peony, tangkuei.

COPTIS TOXIN-RESOLVING DECOCTION

Ōrengedokutō   huáng lián jiĕ dú tāng

COMPOSITION

| coptis | 1.5-2g. | phellodendron | 1.5-3g. |
| scutellaria | 3g. | gardenia | 2-3g. |

PATTERN

Constitutional state   (5 4 3) 2 1

Typical traits/predisposing factors
Habitus apoplecticus with ruddy complexion

Signs and symptoms

Heat .... • headrush syndrome – associated symptoms include flushing, headaches, ocular rubor, palpitations, dizziness, tinnitus

• hyperemic or inflammatory conditions in general

• psychologic symptoms such as irritability, insomnia, restlessness, anxiety; possibly manic agitation or delirium in severe cases

• thirst, bad breath, bitter taste in the mouth

Others .... • distress in the upper abdomen or chest

• acute bleeding (blood that is relatively bright red in color)

Abdominal findings .... • possibly, an unusual warmth may be palpable in the center of the chest, and points on the anterior midline over the sternum may be tender to pressure

TCM pattern identification
Exuberant heat, blood heat, damp-heat, effulgent heart and liver fire

---

APPLICATIONS

Hot flushes and other vasomotor manifestations

Sleep disturbances .... •especially suitable for difficulty in initiating sleep

• can also be beneficial for difficulty in maintaining sleep or dream-troubled sleep; may be even more effective in combination with Counterflow Cold Powder if indications exist

Emotional distress .... • anxiety, depression, neurotic conditions

Abnormal bleeding/menstrual disorders/vaginal symptoms ....
- • dysfunctional uterine bleeding, menorrhagia, polymenorrhea

Urinary disorders ....
- • may be applied in acute cystourethritis when there is bleeding and marked inflammation

Hypertension, hyperlipidemia, atherosclerosis ....
- • tend to be suitable for persons with "A-type" personality
- • may be combined with a bupleurum formula if indications exist
- • also useful as a preventative for stroke and in long term treatment for myocardial infarction and angina

ADDITIONAL APPLICATIONS

GI..
- • stomatitis, acute gastroenteritis, chronic gastritis, peptic ulcer (can be highly effective for bleeding due to these conditions)

Skin ....
- • eczema, urticaria, acne, psoriasis, sunburn

Bleeding ....
- • hematemesis, nosebleed, hemoptysis, bleeding from the eye, bleeding hemorrhoids

Others ....
- • hangover, vicarious menstruation (commonly in the form of nosebleed), acute infectious disorders, psychotic disorders, dementia

NOTES

Generally to be taken with cool water.

May be combined with other formulas to provide additional "cooling" actions for marked heat symptoms, such as acute inflammations or morbidly excited states.

Add rhubarb in cases with tendency to constipation. The dose should be adjusted to achieve regular bowel movements. Alternatively, prescribe Three Yellows Heart-Draining Decoction. The pattern and applications of the latter formula are similar to those for Coptis Toxin-Resolving Decoction, with tendency to constipation as an additional feature.

Can have a drying effect on the body in long-term use. Consider Warm Clearing Beverage for chronic inflammatory or bleeding conditions, or if the symptom picture includes signs of blood vacuity (e.g., dry lusterless skin).

Very bitter-tasting, but the taste tends to be well tolerated by patients manifesting the above pattern.

Substances on the Caution List: coptis, gardenia.

COUNTERFLOW COLD POWDER

Shigyakusan   *sì nì săn*

COMPOSITION

bupleurum	2-5g.	unripe bitter orange	2g.
peony	2-4g.	licorice	1-2g.

PATTERN

Constitutional state   (5 4 3) 2 1

Signs and symptoms

Psychologic symptoms .... • tension (typically directed inward), depressed mood, insomnia, sense of fatigue

GI disturbances .... • pain or bloating

• difficult bowel movement (thin/pellet-like stool, sense of incomplete evacuation, constipation or constipation alternating with diarrhea)

• nausea

Others .... • excessive muscle tension (neck and shoulder stiffness, tension or abnormal movement in the involuntary muscles)

• cold clammy hands

Abdominal findings .... • <u>subcostal distress</u>

• <u>upper or general rectus tension</u>

• substernal hard glomus

TCM pattern identification

Binding depression of liver qi, liver-spleen disharmony, liver-stomach disharmony

APPLICATIONS

Sleep disturbances .... • difficulty in initiating or maintaining sleep

Emotional distres .... • depression, anxiety, neurotic conditions (including gastrointestinal and psychosexual neuroses)

Chronic headache .... • tension headaches

Abnormal bleeding/menstrual disorders/vaginal symptoms ....

• may be useful in PMS, irregular menstruation or dysmenorrhea

Body aches and pains .... • may be beneficial for stiffness and pain in the neck and shoulder area

ADDITIONAL APPLICATIONS

GI .... • chronic gastroenteritis, gastric hyperacidity, peptic ulcer, colitis, irritable bowel syndrome, nervous abdominal pains, esophageal spasm, reflux esophagitis

Hepato-biliary..................... • gallstones, inflammation of the gallbladder, chronic hepatitis

Others............................... •nephritis, nephrosis, hypertension, paraplegia, rhinitis, sinusitis, bronchitis, bronchial asthma

NOTES

The GI symptoms result in part from abnormal peristalsis. This formula may be beneficial in dysfunctions associated with excessive tone or spasms of the smooth muscles. Examples include spastic colon and spasms of the pylorus.

May be combined with Coptis Toxin-Resolving Decoction if indications exist (e.g., red face and marked irritability). A small amount of Counterflow Cold Powder may also be added to various formulas to treat dysphoria accompanying chronic illness.

Substances on the Caution List: licorice, peony, unripe bitter orange.

CYPERUS AND PERILLA POWDER

Kōsosan   *xiāng sū sǎn*

COMPOSITION

cyperus	3.5-6g.	tangerine peel	2-3g.	dried ginger	1-2g.
perilla leaf	1-2g.	licorice	1.-1.5g.		

PATTERN

Constitutional state   5 (4 3 2) 1

Signs and symptoms

Psychologic symptoms .... • pent-up tension, unvented feelings, depressed mood

GI symptoms .... • feeling of distension

• pain (characteristically varies in intensity or location and can be related to emotional changes)

• nausea, vomiting

• loss of appetite

Others .... • headaches, heavy-headedness

• dizziness

Abdominal findings .... • substernal hard glomus

TCM pattern identification

Qi stagnation (spleen-stomach qi stagnation), exterior cold with qi stagnation

APPLICATIONS

Emotional distress .... • depression, nervous abdominal pain, GI neurosis and other neurotic conditions, premenstrual tension, unresolved stress reactions, etc.

Chronic headaches

Abnormal bleeding/menstrual disorders/vaginal symptoms ....

• psychogenic dysmenorrhea or amenorrhea

ADDITIONAL APPLICATIONS

Initial stage of common cold (at the very first sign), skin rash or urticaria due to fish or other food poisoning

NOTES

This formula is rich in essential oils that are likely to be lost in the usual extract manufacture process. Dosage increase may thus be necessary with extract preparations.

An efficacious as well as convenient alternative is to mix the powdered herbs directly with some hot water. In this case, the daily dosage should be 2/3 of the dosage given above. A hot decoction of scallion (the root and white part of 2-5 scallions) instead of plain water would make it even more potent.

Substances on the Caution List: ginger, licorice, perilla leaf.

Contraindication: Because of the aromatic, drying and dispersive nature of this formula, it should be used cautiously and only for a short term in cases complicated by fluid deficiency (yin vacuity); or by a lack, and not merely a stagnation, of vital energy (qi vacuity). Do not prescribe if either condition is marked.

EIGHT-INGREDIENT DISCHARGE FORMULA

Hachimitaigehō   *bā wèi dài xià fāng*

COMPOSITION

tangkuei	5g.	poria	3g.	lonicera	1g.
smooth greenbrier	4g.	mutong	3g.	rhubarb	0.3-1g.
ligusticum	3g.	tangerine peel	2g.		

PATTERN

Constitutional state   5 (4 3 2) 1

Signs and symptoms

Abnormal vaginal discharge

Others .... • itching in the genital area

• constipation

• lower abdominal pain

Abdominal findings .... • mild blood stasis signs

TCM pattern identification

Damp-heat

APPLICATIONS

Abnormal bleeding/menstrual disorders/vaginal symptoms ....

• abnormal vaginal discharge, vaginitis, atrophic vaginitis

ADDITIONAL APPLICATIONS

Gynecologic .... • vaginal discharge associated with venereal disease

NOTES

Broadly applicable in cases without marked inflammation. May be combined with blood stasis formulas.

Discontinue use if diarrhea occurs and persists; or if possible, prescribe without rhubarb.

Not as commonly available in extract format.

Substances on the Caution List: ligusticum, mutong, tangkuei, *rhubarb.

EIGHT-INGREDIENT REHMANNIA PILLS

Hachimijiōgan   *bā wèi dì huáng wán*

COMPOSITION

rehmannia	5-8g.	alisma	3g.	cinnamon twig	1g.
cornus	3-4g.	poria	3g.	processed aconite	0.5-1g.
dioscorea	3-4g.	moutan	3g.		

PATTERN

Constitutional state   5 4 (3 2 1)

Signs and symptoms

Conditions marked by <u>degenerative changes and decline in functions</u>, commonly associated with aging and generally involving one or more of the underlined indications:

<u>Limpness or pain in the lumbar region or knees</u>

Cold/Heat .... • cold sensitivity

• cold lumbar region or cold extremities (more evident in cold weather); may be accompanied by heat in the palms and soles (more evident in warm weather)

Fluid imbalance .... • abnormal micturition

• mouth dryness or thirst with preference for warm drinks

• mild edema

Others .... • easy fatigability

• numbness, tingling

• impaired vision

• tinnitus, impaired hearing

• decline in mental abilities

• dry itchy skin

• shortness of breath

Abdominal finding .... • <u>hypotonic lower abdomen</u>

• <u>lower rectus tension</u>

TCM pattern identification

Kidney yang vacuity, kidney yin-yang dual vacuity

APPLICATIONS

Abnormal bleeding/menstrual disorders/vaginal symptoms ....
- abnormal vaginal discharge, itching of the external genitals, atrophic vaginitis

Urinary disorders .... • abnormal micturition, including polyuria, oliguria, nocturia, dysuria, frequency, hesitancy, postvoid dribbling, sense of incomplete voiding and incontinence

- applicable in chronic or recurrent cystourethritis, urethral syndrome, other disorders not explained by urologic findings, incontinence

Body aches and pains, osteoporosis ....
- chronic low back pain, sciatica
- may be beneficial in osteoporosis and other degenerative disorders of the bone

Hypertension, hyperlipidemia, atherosclerosis

ADDITIONAL APPLICATIONS

Nervous .... • neuritis, neuralgia, neuropathy, weakness or paralysis of the lower limbs

EENT .... • cataract, glaucoma, floaters

Skin .... • prurigo senilis, eczema, psoriasis

Urinary .... • renal disorders such as chronic nephritis, nephrosis, urinary calculi

Others .... • diabetes mellitus, chronic constipation in the elderly, congestive heart failure, low blood pressure, senile dementia, hypothyroidism, impotence, prostatitis, hypertrophy of the prostate

NOTES

The abdominal findings – hypotonic lower abdomen and lower rectus tension – may occur singly, but the two most often occur together. Both may be prominent; or there may be a marked softness in the middle with mild degree of rectus tension; or conversely, somewhat soft middle with marked rectus tension. The resulting impression is that of a central softness sandwiched between tenseness.

Age is a contributing but not determining factor in the application of this formula

Useful in a wide variety of disorders which tend to affect older adults, alone or as an adjunct. May minimize the impact of aging-related changes.

Can be more effective than conventional drug therapy in controlling and preventing complications of diabetes such as peripheral neuropathy, nephropathy, and retinopathy.

See Prevention of GI Disturbances, p. 85. If so desired, this formula may be taken with a little alcohol to aid digestion and assimilation, and to augment its efficacy.

Substances on the Caution List: *aconite, cinnamon, moutan, *rehmannia.

Contraindications: Diarrhea, anorexia.

When the patient has gastrointestinal problems, consider formulas such as Cinnamon Twig Decoction Plus Atractylodes and Aconite, True Warrior Decoction, Ginseng Decoction, Bupleurum, Cinnamon Twig and Dried Ginger Decoctionm, or Heart-Clearing Lotus Seed Beverage.

Related Formulas

• **Achyranthes and Plantago Kidney Qi Pills**

Composed of Eight-Ingredient Rehmannia Pills with the addition of achyranthes and plantago.

Indicated in cases with more marked edema, oliguria, lower back pain, weakness in the lumbar region or knees, or impairment of vision (glaucoma, retinopathy). May be tried if Eight-Ingredient Rehmannia Pills is ineffective.

Substances on the Caution List: achyranthes, *aconite, cinnamon, moutan, *rehmannia.

• **Six-Ingredient Rehmannia Pills**

Eight-Ingredient Rehmannia Pills formulated without cinnamon and aconite.

This formula is more suitable if the pattern neither includes cold signs (cold extremities, cold sensitivity) nor edema, but has more pronounced heat signs (thirst for cold drinks, heat in the palms or soles, generalized heat sensation, headrushes/flushing, irritability and insomnia).

TCM pattern identification: kidney yin vacuity.

Substances on the Caution List: moutan, *rehmannia.

EVODIA DECOCTION

Goshuyutō   *wú zhū yú tāng*

COMPOSITION

evodia	3-4g.	jujube	3-6g.
ginseng	2-3g.	fresh ginger	4-6g.

PATTERN

Constitutional state   5 4 3 (2 1)

Signs and symptoms

Fluid imbalance (in conjunction with Cold) ....
- attacks of severe headaches
- dizziness
- retching or vomiting, often with marked nausea
- oppressive discomfort in the chest and upper abdomen
- excessive salivation

Coldness syndrome ....• cold extremities, especially during an attack

Others ....• headrush (facial flushing) during an attack

Abdominal findings .... • substernal hard glomus (distention during an attack)
- substernal splashing sound
- periumbilical pulsation

TCM pattern identification

Counterflow ascent of cold rheum, stomach vacuity cold

APPLICATIONS

Chronic headaches ....• a typical attack is characterized by muscular tightness affecting the neck and extending up to the temple(s) (may be unilateral or bilateral); distress in the chest and epigastric region; and cold extremities; marked nausea, vomiting, and agitation may accompany a severe attack; fatigue, dietary indiscretion, or premenstrual tension are common triggering factors
- may be applied in migraines, headaches with nausea and vomiting, headaches associated with PMS, etc.

ADDITIONAL APPLICATIONS

Nausea and vomiting, gastritis, peptic ulcer, food/drug poisoning, hiccups

NOTES

Although bitter and strong-tasting, this formula tends to be well-tolerated by patients exhibiting the above pattern.

Will also alleviate symptoms during an attack (to be taken little by little in small sips).

Substances on the Caution List: evodia, ginger, ginseng, jujube.

FANGJI AND ASTRAGALUS DECOCTION
Bōiōgitō   *fāng jǐ huáng qí tāng*

COMPOSITION

| fangji | 4-5g. | ovate atractylodes | 3g. | jujube | 3-4g. |
| astragalus | 5g. | fresh ginger | 3g. | licorice | 1.5-2g. |

PATTERN

Constitutional state   5 4 (3 2) 1

Typical traits/predisposing factors
tendency to be puffy and overweight

Signs and symptoms

Asthenia .... • tendency to spontaneous sweating
• flaccid adipose flesh
• easy fatigability
• shortness of breath
• aversion to wind

Fluid imbalance .... • reduced urinary output
• edema (esp. in the lower limbs)
• sense of heaviness and laborious movement
• swollen and painful joint (esp. the knee)

Abdominal findings .... • typically rounded contour with poor muscle tone

TCM pattern identification
Wind-damp (or wind water or water swelling) and qi vacuity

APPLICATIONS

Abnormal bleeding/menstrual disorders/vaginal symptoms ....
• menstrual disorders

Body aches and pains, osteoporosis ....
• all chronic rheumatic conditions without evident
heat and rubor, esp. swollen and painful knees.
combination with Spleen-Effusing Decoction
Plus Ovate Atractylodes or Coix Decoction
may be considered for cases with heat and more
acute pain in the affected part
• may be beneficial in osteoporosis

Hypertension, atherosclerosis, obesity

ADDITIONAL APPLICATIONS

Urinary .... • nephritis, nephrosis, toxemia of pregnancy

Skin .... • urticaria, dermatitis, pyogenic conditions of the lower limbs, excessive perspiration

Others .... • neuralgia, gout, edema, obesity

NOTES

Substances on the Caution List: ginger, jujube, licorice.

FIVE ACCUMULATIONS POWDER

Goshakusan   *wŭ jī săn*

COMPOSITION

poria	2g.	ligusticum	1-2g.	cinnamon twig	1-2g.
ovate atractylodes	3-4g.	magnolia bark	1-2g.	ephedra	1-2g.
tangerine peel	2g.	angelica	1-2g.	jujube	1-2g.
pinellia	2g.	unripe bitter orange	1-2g.	licorice	1-2g.
tangkuei	1.5-2g.	platycodon	1-2g.	cyperus	0/1.2g.
peony	1-2g.	dried ginger	1-2g.		

(None or up to 1.2g of cyperus can be used.)

PATTERN

Constitutional state   5 (4 3 2) 1

Signs and symptoms

Cold/heat .... • <u>symptoms precipitated or aggravated by cold or cold and damp</u> in the environment, or overconsumption of raw and cold foods

• upper body heat and lower body cold (associated symptoms include headrushes, flushing or unusual warmth in the upper body without perspiration, headaches, cold lower body and lower extremities); or possibly just cold lower body and lower extremities

• aches and pains associated with coldness (esp. in the abdomen, lower back or thighs)

GI disturbances (related to coldness and fluid imbalance) ....

• abdominal discomfort or pain

• nausea, vomiting

• diarrhea

Blood imbalance .... • menstrual disorders

Abdominal finding .... • substernal hard glomus

• blood stasis signs

TCM pattern identification

Cold damp, exterior-interior cold, channel and connecting vessels cold stroke or visceral cold stroke

APPLICATIONS

Chronic headaches

Abnormal bleeding/menstrual disorders/vaginal symptoms ....
- irregular menstruation, dysmenorrhea, abnormal vaginal discharge

Body aches and pains, osteoporosis ....
- arthritis, low back pain, sciatica (esp. with stiffness and coldness in the sacrum area), fibrositis
- may be beneficial in osteoporosis

ADDITIONAL APPLICATIONS

GI .... • peptic ulcer, gastric spasms, gastroenteritis

Others .... • neuralgia, hemiplegia (stroke), recurrent cystitis, common cold, influenza, overexposure to air conditioning

NOTES

See note on ephedra in Appendix A. To minimize the possibility of adverse effects from misuse of this formula, start with a small dose or have the patient take it after eating.

Substances on the Caution List: cinnamon, *ephedra, ginger, jujube, licorice, ligusticum, magnolia bark, peony, pinellia, tangkuei, unripe bitter orange.

FIVE STRANGURIES POWDER

Gorinsan   *wŭ lín săn*

COMPOSITION

Six ingredient:

poria	5-6g.	scutellaria	3g.	peony	2g.
tangkuei	3g.	licorice	3g.	gardenia	2g.

Eleven ingredient:

poria	5-6g.	peony	2g.	mutong	3g.
tangkuei	3g.	gardenia	2g.	talcum	3g.
scutellaria	3g.	rehmannia	3g.	plantago seed	3g.
licorice	3g.	alisma	3g.		

PATTERN

Constitutional state   (5 4 3 2) 1

Signs and symptoms

Inflammatory conditions of the lower urinary tract..

  •symptoms such as dysuria, frequency, concentrated
  urine, sense of incomplete voiding, blood or pus
  in the urine

TCM pattern identification

The five stranguries: qi strangury, calculous strangury, blood strangury,
unctuous strangury, taxation strangury

APPLICATIONS

Urinary disorders ....•cystourethritis, urethral syndrome and other
  disorders not explained by urologic findings,
  incontinence associated with irritative symptoms
  •may also relieve low-grade back pain associated
  with chronic conditions.

ADDITIONAL APPLICATIONS

Urinary calculi, gonorrhea

NOTES

This is a general formula for urinary complaints that can be tried in all cases without marked inflammation. It is somewhat superior in diuretic action to Gentian
Liver-Draining Decoction (the *Sesshi* version), while the latter has a somewhat
stronger anti-inflammatory effect.

Can be very effective for oliguria with dysuria or sense of incomplete voiding associated with excessive sweating in hot weather.

The composition differs depending on the historical source. The six- and eleven-ingredient versions, common in Japanese extract preparations, are given above. The more complex formulation incorporates additional anti-inflammatory and diuretic actions.

Substances on the Caution List: gardenia, *licorice, peony, tangkuei (mutong, *rehmannia).

FREEING ABDUCTION POWDER

Tsūdōsan   *tōng dǎo sǎn*

COMPOSITION

tangkuei	3g.	magnolia bark	2g.	sappan	2g.
rhubarb	3g.	tangerine peel	2g.	licorice	2g.
mirabilite	3-4g.	mutong	2g.		
unripe bitter orange	2-3g.	carthamus	2g.		

PATTERN

Constitutional state   (5 4) 3 2 1

Signs and symptoms
Blood stasis conditions

Others .... • feeling of distention in the lower abdomen or
generalized distention

• tendency to constipation

• symptoms secondary to impaired circulation, such
as headaches, dizziness, neck and shoulder stiffness

Abdominal findings .... • blood stasis signs
distention

TCM pattern identification
Blood stasis with qi stagnation

APPLICATIONS

Abnormal bleeding/menstrual disorders/vaginal symptoms ....
• dysfunctional uterine bleeding, irregular
menstruation, dysmenorrhea, PMS, vaginitis

Urinary disorders ....
• may be applied in conditions with the above pattern

Body aches and pains, osteoporosis ....
• low back pain, sciatica, fibrositis

• may be beneficial in osteoporosis

Hypertension, hyperlipidemia, atherosclerosis

ADDITIONAL APPLICATIONS

Sprains, impact trauma (bruise, internal bleeding, urinary retention, etc.), pelvic
infection, hemiplegia

NOTES

Created originally to treat acute trauma.

This formula may be applied much like Peach Kernel Qi-Infusing Decoction, although it is not as widely employed in present-day Japan. Peach kernel and moutan are often added to heighten its efficacy. With extracts, this may be achieved by combination with Cinnamon Twig and Poria Pills.

Substances on the Caution List: carthamus, licorice, magnolia bark, *mirabilite, mutong, *rhubarb, sappan, tangkuei, unripe bitter orange.

GENTIAN LIVER-DRAINING DECOCTION

Ryūtanshakantō   *lóng dǎn xiè gān tāng*

COMPOSITION

Nine ingredient *(Sesshi)*

tangkuei	5g.	alisma	3g.	licorice	1-1.5g.
rehmannia	5g.	plantago seed	3g.		
mutong	5g.	gentian	1-1.5g.		
scutellaria	3g.	gardenia	1-1.5g.		

Sixteen ingredient *(Ikkandō)*

tangkuei	1.5g.	phellodendron	1.5g.	plantago seed	1.5g.
peony	1.5g.	gardenia	1.5g.	licorice	1.5g.
ligusticum	1.5g.	forsythia	1.5g.	gentian	2g.
rehmannia	1.5g.	mint leaf	1.5g.	alisma	2g.
coptis	1.5g.	mutong	1.5g.		
scutellaria	1.5g.	ledebouriella	1.5g.		

PATTERN

Constitutional state   (5 4 3) 2 1

Signs and symptoms

Inflammatory conditions of the lower urinary tract or the reproductive apparatus,

- symptoms include hyperemia, swelling, pain, burning or itching

Abdominal findings .... • tension and tenderness along the lateral borders of the recti (more precisely, along the acupuncture liver channel)

TCM pattern identification

Damp-heat in the lower burner

APPLICATIONS

Abnormal bleeding/menstrual disorders/vaginal symptoms ....

- vaginitis, atrophic vaginitis

Urinary disorders .... • cystourethritis, urethral syndrome and other disorders not explained by urologic findings, incontinence associated with irritative symptoms

- may also relieve low-grade back pain associated with chronic conditions

ADDITIONAL APPLICATIONS

Gynecologic .... • pelvic inflammatory disease, bartholinitis, genital eczema

Others .... • gonorrhea, urinary calculi, hemorrhoids

NOTES

Two formulations are current in Japan. The *Sesshi* version, commonly available in extract format, has stronger anti-inflammatory effects and is usually for short term use in acute to subacute conditions. The more complex *Ikkandō* version is suitable for chronic or recurrent conditions and can be used over a longer time period as a constitutional alterative.

See note under Five Stranguries Powder.

Substances on the Caution List: gardenia, licorice, mutong, *rehmannia, tangkuei (coptis, ledebouriella, ligusticum, peony).

GINSENG DECOCTION

Ninjintō   *rén shēn tāng*

COMPOSITION

ginseng	3g.	ovate atractylodes	3g.
licorice	3g.	dried ginger	2-3g.

PATTERN

Constitutional state   5 4 3 (2 1)

Signs and symptoms

Coldness syndrome .... •cold sensitivity (acute GI symptoms may be precipitated by exposure to cold or excessive consumption of cold foods and drinks

• cold extremities, cold abdomen

• long voidings of clear urine, frequent urination

Weak digestive function .... • poor appetite

• substernal discomfort

• bloating or pain

• excessive salivation or mouth dryness

• nausea, vomiting

• tendency to diarrhea (less commonly, constipation)

• sluggishness or drowsiness after eating

Others .... • general feeling of tiredness

• oppression or pain in the chest

Abdominal findings .... • substernal hard glomus (or hypotonicity)

• substernal splashing sound (or less commonly, general rectus tension)

• hypotonic lower abdomen

TCM pattern identification

Spleen-stomach yang vacuity, or direct strike of center by cold pathogen

---

APPLICATIONS

Body aches and pains, osteoporosis ....

• may be beneficial in cases of shoulder stiffness or pain with the above pattern

• may be useful in osteoporosis (normalizes the GI function)

ADDITIONAL APPLICATIONS

GI .... • dyspepsia, gastritis, gastric atony, peptic ulcer, irritable bowel syndrome, ulcerative colitis, diarrhea after abdominal surgery

Others .... • anemia, infertility, vomiting in pregnancy, diabetes, intercostal neuralgia, heart disorders, hypothyroidism

NOTES

May be useful in reducing the GI sides effects of drugs.

If edema occurs during administration of this formula, it generally signals misuse or overdosage. Reconsider the pattern. Poria Five Powder can be used to treat the edema.

Substances on the Caution List: ginger, ginseng, *licorice.

GODDESS POWDER

Nyoshinsan   *nǚ shén sǎn*

COMPOSITION

tangkuei	3-4g.	scutellaria	2-4g.	clove	0.5-1g.
ligusticum	3g.	ginseng	1.5-2g.	licorice	1-1.5g.
ovate atractylodes	3g.	areca seed	2-4g.	rhubarb	0/0.5-1g.
cyperus	3-4g.	coptis	1-2g.		
cinnamon twig	2-3g.	saussurea	1-2g.		

(None or up to 0.5-1 g. of rhubarb can be used.)

PATTERN

Constitutional state   (5 4 3) 2 1

Signs and symptoms

Psychologic symptoms .... • depressed mood, anxiety, insomnia

Headrush syndrome .... • headrushes (flushes)
                                      • dizziness
                                      • heavy-headedness, headaches
                                      • palpitations

Others .... • abdominal distress (symptoms such as distention
                                       or pain, nausea) or sense of oppression in the chest
                                      • menstrual disorders
                                      • sense of fatigue

Abdominal findings .... • substernal hard glomus
                                      • blood stasis signs
                                      • periumbilical pulsation

TCM pattern identification

Qi stagnation with signs of qi-blood dual vacuity and effulgent heart and liver fire

APPLICATIONS

Hot flushes and other vasomotor manifestations

Sleep disturbances .... • difficulty in initiating sleep

Emotional distress .... • depression, anxiety, nervous symptoms associated
                                    with hormonal fluctuation (premenstrual tension,
                                    pre- and postpartum or menopausal neuroses),
                                    other neurotic conditions

Chronic headaches

Abnormal bleeding/menstrual disorders/vaginal symptoms ....
• irregular menstruation, dysmenorrhea, PMS

Hypertension .... • may be beneficial in cases of hypertension in the perimenopause showing the above pattern

NOTES

Originally created to treat neurotic conditions in soldiers fighting in the front.

Prescribe without rhubarb in cases without tendency to constipation.

Substances on the Caution List: cinnamon, coptis, ginseng, licorice, ligusticum, tangkuei (*rhubarb)

HEART-CLEARING LOTUS SEED BEVERAGE
Seishinrenshiin   *qīng xīn lián zǐ yǐn*

COMPOSITION

lotus seed	4g.	ginseng	3g.	astragalus	2g.
ophiopogon	4g.	plantago seed	3g.	lycium root bark	2g.
poria	4g.	scutellaria	3g.	licorice	1.5-2g.

PATTERN

Constitutional state   5 4 (3 2 1)

Signs and symptoms

<u>Chronic lower urinary tract problems</u> (little evidence of inflammation), with symptoms such as frequency, dysuria, cloudy urine, concentrated urine, sense of incomplete voiding, poor stream, incontinence; associated with one or both of the following:

1. Psychologic symptoms – such as excessive worry, vexation, disturbed sleep
2. Asthenia – feeling of tiredness, easy fatigability, poor appetite (or weak digestive function)

Others ....• mouth or throat dryness
• heat sensation in the palms or soles
• abnormal vaginal discharge
Abdominal findings .... • substernal hard glomus

TCM pattern identification

Qi and yin dual vacuity with vacuity fire of the heart, upper body exuberance and lower body vacuity

APPLICATIONS

Abnormal bleeding/menstrual disorders/vaginal symptoms ....
• abnormal vaginal discharge, atrophic vaginitis
Urinary disorders .... • applicable in chronic or recurrent cystourethritis, psychogenic urinary frequency, urethral syndrome and other disorders not explained by urologic findings; incontinence

ADDITIONAL APPLICATIONS

Urinary calculi, chronic pyelitis, gonorrhea, stomatitis

NOTES

Also applicable in sleep disturbances (difficulty in initiating or maintaining sleep, dream-troubled sleep) and neurotic conditions in individuals with the above asthenic signs and urinary problems.

To be taken with cold water if the heat symptoms are pronounced.

Substances on the Caution List: ginseng, licorice.

HONEY-FRIED LICORICE DECOCTION

Shakanzōtō   *zhì gān cǎo tāng*

COMPOSITION

licorice	3-4g.	hemp seed	3g.	rehmannia	4-6g.
fresh ginger	1-3g.	jujube	3-5g.	ophiopogon	6g.
cinnamon twig	3g.	ginseng	2-3g.	ass hide glue	2g.

PATTERN

Constitutional state   5 4 3 (2 1)

Signs and symptoms

<u>Cardiac palpitations</u>, accompanied by breathlessness, oppression or pain in the chest, possibly also arrhythmia.

Asthenia .... • feeling of tiredness, easy fatigability
                                  • night sweating
Heat .... • tendency to headrushes (flushing)
                                  • sensation of heat in the extremities
                                  • restlessness, poor sleep
Others (dryness) .... • dry skin
                                  • mouth dryness
                                  • tendency to constipation
Abdominal findings .... • periumbilical pulsation

TCM pattern identification

Qi and yin dual vacuity of the heart

APPLICATIONS

Emotional distress .... • applicable in cardiac neurosis and other neurotic
                                  conditions with the above pattern

ADDITIONAL APPLICATIONS

Hyperactivity of the sympathetic nervous system, hyperthyroidism, heart disorders (ectopic beats, valve disorders, heart block, etc.), pulmonary tuberculosis, diabetes mellitus, hypertension

NOTES

Substances on the Caution List: cinnamon, ginger, ginseng, jujube, *licorice, *rehmannia

Contraindication: Not suitable if the patient has weak digestive function or experiences diarrhea from the use of this formula.

LEDEBOURIELLA SAGE-INSPIRED POWDER

Bōfūtsūshōsan   *fáng fēng tōng shèng sǎn*

COMPOSITION

tangkuei	1.2g.	fresh ginger	1.2g.	ovate atractylodes	2g.
peony	1.2g.	schizonepeta	1.2g.	platycodon	2g.
ligusticum	1.2g.	ledebouriella	1.2g.	scutellaria	2g.
charred gardenia	1.2g.	ephedra	1.2g.	licorice	2g.
forsythia	1.2g.	rhubarb	1.5g.	gypsum	2-3g.
mint leaf	1.2g.	mirabilite	1.5g.	talcum	3-5g.

PATTERN

Constitutional state   (5 4 3) 2 1

Typical traits/predisposing factors

Habitus apoplecticus

Signs and symptoms

Sthenia and Heat .... • signs of caloric excess

• tendency to constipation

• headrush syndrome – associated symptoms such as flushing, headaches, neck and shoulder stiffness, ocular rubor, thirst, tinnitus, palpitations, insomnia

• tendency toward skin problems (e.g., seborrheic dermatitis)

• dark-colored urine

Abdominal findings .... • typically firm abdomen with rounded contour (excessive subcutaneous fat)

TCM pattern identification

Wind heat, exterior cold and interior repletion heat

APPLICATIONS

Hot flushes and other vasomotor manifestations

Urinary disorders .... • may be beneficial in cystitis and other inflammatory or irritative conditions

Hypertension, hyperlipidemia, atherosclerosis ....

• relieves symptoms that commonly accompany hypertension

ADDITIONAL APPLICATIONS

Hormonal-metabolic .... • diabetes mellitus, gout

Skin .... • eczema, urticaria, boils, rosacea, erysipelas, excessive hair loss

EENT .... • otorrhea, partial hearing loss, sinusitis

Others .... • constipation, hemorrhoids, venereal disease, influenza, bronchitis

NOTES

Ledebouriella Sage-Inspired Powder, originally used for acute febrile or inflammatory conditions, is employed in present-day Kampo mainly as a constitutional alterative for various chronic disorders. It can be suitable for individuals without an obvious protruding abdomen.

This formula promotes elimination through diaphoresis and through the urinary and digestive tracts. It also ameliorates inflammatory conditions and has a favorable effect on lipid metabolism. As such, it is useful as an alterative in hypertension, atherosclerosis and obesity, and can be considered in long-term treatment of angina pectoris, myocardial infarction or stroke, to lower risks of future attacks.

Substances on the Caution List: *ephedra, gardenia, ginger, gypsum, ledebouriella, licorice, ligusticum, *mirabilite, peony, *rhubarb, schizonepeta, tangkuei.

LICORICE HEART-DRAINING DECOCTION

Kanzōshashintō   *gān cǎo xiè xīn tāng*

COMPOSITION

pinellia	4-5g.	jujube	2.5g.	coptis	1g.
dried ginger	2-2.5g.	scutellaria	2.5-3g.		
ginseng	2.5g.	licorice	3-4.5g.		

NOTES

See under Pinellia Heart-Draining Decoction.

Substances on the Caution List: coptis, ginger, ginseng, jujube, *licorice, pinellia.

LICORICE, WHEAT AND JUJUBE DECOCTION
Kanbakutaisōtō   *gān mài dà zăo tāng*

COMPOSITION

licorice	5g.	jujube	6g.
light wheat grain	20g.		

PATTERN

Constitutional state   5 (4 3 2) 1

Signs and symptoms

Psychologic symptoms .... • tearfulness, sadness, anxiety, hysteric fits of crying or laughing, insomnia, marked excitement

Asthenia .... • frequent yawning (esp. after a hysteric fit)
• easy fatigability

Others .... • spasms/convulsions
• hyperventilation
• fainting

Abdominal findings .... • general rectus tension, esp. at the right side periumbilical pulsation

TCM pattern identification

Visceral agitation, heart blood vacuity

APPLICATIONS

Sleep disturbances .... • difficulty in initiating or maintaing sleep, nonrestorative sleep, dream-troubled sleep (night terrors)

Emotional distress .... • hysteria, anxiety, depression, neurotic conditions

ADDITIONAL APPLICATIONS

Chorea, epilepsy, tics, somnambulism, hyperventilation, manic-depressive illness, anorexia nervosa, uterine spasm, gastric spasm

NOTES

This formula may be taken regularly or on an as-needed basis.

The decoction is preferable. Wheat being an ingredient, extract preparations of this formula would either be weak or chemically altered (such as through caramelization). On the other hand, the syrup of this formula is effective, can be prepared in advance, and keeps well in the refrigerator. It may be made by simmering the 3 ingredients in water (about 1/2 quart per daily dosage specified above; use crushed whole wheat kernels) until reduced to the consistency of a syrup. Strain and refrigerate. Dilute and heat through before taking.

Substances on the Caution List: jujube, *licorice.

LIGUSTICUM, TANGKUEI, ASS HIDE GLUE AND MUGWORT DECOCTION
Kyūkikyōgaitō   *xiōng guī jiāo ài tāng*

COMPOSITION

ligusticum	3g.	ass hide glue	3g.	rehmannia	5g.
artemisia	3g.	licorice	3g.		
peony	4-4.5g.	tangkuei	4-4.5g.		

PATTERN

Constitutional state   5 4 (3 2 1)

Signs and symptoms

Blood imbalance .... • bleeding or tendency to bleed, especially from the lower half of the body (often in the form of continual loss of small amount of blood)

• blood vacuity or anemia

Others .... • pain or numbness in the lower abdomen

Abdominal findings .... • softness

• blood stasis signs

• periumbilical pulsation

• lower rectus tension, esp. at the left

TCM pattern identification

Bleeding and blood vacuity

APPLICATIONS

Abnormal bleeding/menstrual disorders/vaginal symptoms ....

• abnormal uterine bleeding, especially long-term bleeding problems, i.e., menorrhagia, dysfunctional uterine bleeding, bleeding associated with fibroids, excessive or unusual post-surgical bleeding.

ADDITIONAL APPLICATIONS

Gynecologic .... • threatened abortion, excessive or unusual postpartum bleeding

Bleeding .... • purpura, hematemesis, intestinal bleeding, hemorrhoidal bleeding, bleeding from the urinary tract, bleeding due to injuries, anemia

NOTES

Frequently prescribed in abnormal uterine bleeding. Quickly arrests bleeding and alleviates anemic conditions.

Also applicable in ordinarily sthenic individuals weakened by chronic or excessive bleeding, childbirth or surgical operations.

See Prevention of GI Disturbances, p. 85. In individuals with weak digestive function or tendency to diarrhea, Spleen-Returning Decoction may be considered instead. Alternatively, try the original version of this formula which contains only the four substances after which it was named: ligusticum, tangkuei, gelatin, and artemisia.

Substances on the Caution List: *licorice, ligusticum, peony, *rehmannia, tangkuei.

Contraindications

• Not suitable for severely anemic conditions.

• Not suitable by itself if heat is a significant feature – i.e., if hyperemia or inflammation, or symptoms such as flushing, thirst for cold drinks or heat intolerance are prominent. Consider formulas such as Channel-Warming Decoction, Warm Clearing Beverage, Cinnamon Twig and Poria Pills, Peach Kernel Qi-Infusing Decoction or Coptis Toxin-Resolving Decoction in such cases.

LIVER-REPRESSING POWDER

Yokukansan   *yì gān sǎn*

COMPOSITION

tangkuei	3g.	ovate atractylodes	4g.	licorice	1.5g.
uncaria	3g.	poria	4g.		
ligusticum	3g.	bupleurum	2g.		

PATTERN

Constitutional state   5 4 (3 2) 1

Signs and symptoms

Psychologic symptoms .... • excitability, impatience, irritability, frequent displays of temper (or tantrums), aggressiveness, insomnia

Excessive muscle tension/involuntary movement ....
- • neck and shoulder stiffness
- • clenching or grinding of the teeth
- • spasms, twitches, tremor, etc.

Others .... • headaches
- • dizziness
- • easy fatigability
- • poor appetite

Abdominal findings .... • tension of the left rectus (generally upper portion); or less commonly, tension in the substernal region
- • mild subcostal distress
- • periumbilical pulsation

TCM pattern identification

Binding depression of liver qi and liver yang transforming into fire, with signs of qi and blood vacuity

APPLICATIONS

Sleep disturbances .... • difficulty in initiating or maintaining sleep, nonrestorative sleep, dream-troubled sleep

Emotional distress .... • anxiety, depression, nervous exhaustion, neurotic conditions

Chronic headaches .... • headaches with the above pattern; may also relieve headaches associated with eyestrain

Hypertension

ADDITIONAL APPLICATIONS

Gynecologic .... • PMS, vomiting in pregnancy

Others .... • stroke (hemiplegia), gout, tics, athetosis, Parkinson's disease, bruxism, epilepsy, trigeminal neuralgia, dementia

NOTES

Can be applied in various disorders of the nervous system featuring the above abdominal signs and involuntary muscle contraction.

Prescribe Liver-Repressing Powder Plus Tangerine Peel and Pinellia instead in cases manifesting prominent abdominal pulsation (possibly also a subjective complaint), or more pronounced signs of fluid stagnancy in the upper abdomen (such as substernal discomfort, bloating or substernal splashing sound).

Substances on the Caution List: licorice, ligusticum, tangkuei (and pinellia in the augmented formulation).

MAJOR BUPLEURUM DECOCTION

Daisaikotō   *dà chái hú tāng*

COMPOSITION

bupleurum	6g.	scutellaria	3g.	unripe bitter orange	2g.
pinellia	3-4g.	white peony	3g.	rhubarb	1-2g.
fresh ginger	4-5g.	jujube	3g.		

PATTERN

Constitutional state   (5 4) 3 2 1

Signs and symptoms

Sthenia ....• mesomorph, wide infrasternal angle

• tendency to constipation

Psychologic symptoms .... • depressed mood, irritability, frequent anger, insomnia

Others ....• distress in the upper abdomen or lateral costal area

• headaches, heavy-headedness

• neck and shoulder stiffness

Abdominal findings .... • <u>marked subcostal distress</u>

• <u>marked substernal hard glomus or distention</u>

(Many other signs and symptoms can be present. Consult "Additional applications.")

TCM pattern identification

Depressed liver qi transforming into fire, liver-stomach disharmony, liver-spleen disharmony

APPLICATIONS

Hot flushes and other vasomotor manifestations

Sleep disturbances

Emotional distress ....• depression, neurotic conditions

Chronic headaches .... • tension headaches, headaches associated with hypertension

Body aches and pains .... • applicable for stiffnesss and pain in the neck and shoulder area

Hypertension, hyperlipidemia, atherosclerosis ....

• tends to be suitable for persons with 'type-A' personality

ADDITIONAL APPLICATIONS

Widely applicable in a variety of diseases:

Respiratory ....• asthma, pleurisy, pulmonary tuberculosis, bronchitis

CV ....• heart diseases, hemorrhoids

GI ....• gastritis, enteritis, peptic ulcer, constipation

Hepato-biliary ....• hepatitis, jaundice, cirrhosis, postoperative liver
problems, gallstones, cholecystitis

Urinary ....• acute and chronic nephritis, nephrosis, urinary calculi

EENT ....• conjunctivitis, iritis, keratitis, cataract, myopia
spuria, otitis media, tinnitus, partial hearing loss,
sinusitis, tonsillitis, pharyngitis, laryngitis

Hormonal-metabolic ....• obesity, diabetes mellitus, gout

Neuromuscular ....• epilepsy, hemiplegia, intercostal neuralgia

Skin ....• urticaria, furuncle, pattern baldness

Others ....• febrile disorders

NOTES

Prescribe without rhubarb (Major Bupleurum Decoction Minus Rhubarb) in cases without tendency to constipation.

Substances on the Caution List: ginger, jujube, peony, pinellia, *rhubarb, unripe bitter orange.

PEACH KERNEL QI-INFUSING DECOCTION
Tōkakujōkitō   *táo hé chéng qì tāng*

COMPOSITION

peach kernel	5g.	raw rhubarb	1-3g.	licorice	1.5g.
cinnamon twig	4g.	mirabilite	1-3g.		

PATTERN

Constitutional state   (5 4) 3 2 1

Signs and symptoms

Blood stasis .... • indications of blood stasis in the pelvic area: menstrual disorders, pelvic congestion syndrome, abnormal genital bleeding, etc.

• other local or general indications of blood stasis

Cold/Heat .... • headrush syndrome – associated symptoms include headaches, neck and shoulder stiffness, dizziness, tinnitus, palpitations, mouth dryness

• cold extremities or lower body (or upper body heat and lower body cold)

• inflammation

Others .... • psychologic symptoms such as anxiety, irritability,
• insomnia, possibly manic agitation or delirium in
• severe cases

• tendency to constipation

Abdominal findings .... • <u>blood stasis signs</u> (esp. in the LLQ)

• LLQ hypersensitivity

TCM pattern identification

Blood stasis, interior repletion heat

APPLICATIONS

Hot flushes and other vasomotor manifestations

Emotional distress .... • symptoms associated with menstrual disorders and other blood stasis conditions; may be applied in neurotic and psychotic conditions.

Chronic headaches .... • tension headaches, headaches associated with menstrual problems and other gynecologic disorders, headaches associated with hypertension or arteriosclerosis

Abnormal bleeding/menstrual disorders/vaginal symptoms ....

• dysfunctional uterine bleeding, dysmenorrhea, irregular menstruation, PMS, vaginitis

- Urinary disorders ....• recurrent cystourethritis, urethral syndrome and other disorders unexplained by urologic findings
- Body aches and pains ......• low back pain, sciatica, fibrositis
  - • may be beneficial in osteoporosis
- Hypertension, arteriosclerosis, hyperlipidemia

ADDITIONAL APPLICATIONS

Gynecologic ....• pelvic inflammatory disease, endometriosis, mastitis, bartholinitis, amenorrhea, infertility, habitual abortion

Skin ....• eczema, urticaria, chilblains, carbuncle, purpura

CV ....• varicose veins, hemorrhoids

Eye ....• blepharitis, iritis, sty

Others ....• bleeding disorders, constipation, urinary calculi, physical injury, epilepsy

NOTES

Like Cinnamon Twig and Poria Pills, this formula is widely used by itself and in combination with other remedies for blood stasis conditions. Whereas the former is in general suitable for cases that are more moderate and settled in manifestation, this formula is called for when symptoms are more severe or more dynamic.

Substances on the Caution List: cinnamon, licorice, *mirabilite, peach kernel, *rhubarb.

PEONY AND LICORICE DECOCTION
Shakuyakukanzōtō   *sháo yào gān cǎo tāng*

COMPOSITION

white peony   3-6g. | honey-fried licorice   3-6g.

PATTERN

Constitutional state   (5 4 3 2 1)

Signs and symptoms

Painful spasms of all smooth and skeletal muscles

Abdominal findings .... • general rectus tension, or any manifestation of tension

APPLICATIONS

Body aches and pains .... • may be applied in back pain, sciatica, arthritis, fibrositis, etc.

ADDITIONAL APPLICATIONS

All conditions featuring spasm and pain; examples include:

Digestive............................ • pain from peptic ulcer, gastritis, intestinal colic, pancreatitis or drug side effect

Urinary .... • urinary calculi (checks attacks of renal and ureteral colic), dysuria

Others .... • painful periods, biliary colic, bronchial asthma, spasmodic cough, hemorrhoidal pain, toothache

ADDITIONAL APPLICATIONS BASED ON RECENT RESEARCH

Anovulation associated with excess blood levels of androgens or prolactin

NOTES

Usually for short term administration, taken as-needed for symptomatic relief.

This remedy can be regarded as the Kampo equivalent of an antispasmodic and non-narcotic analgesic. It is usually used as an adjunct to alleviate acute muscular spasm and pain with another formula that addresses the underlying imbalance.

Substances on the Caution List: *licorice, peony.

PERFECT MAJOR SUPPLEMENTATION DECOCTION
Jyūzentaihotō   *shí quán dà bǔ tāng*

COMPOSITION

ginseng	2.5-3g.	tangkuei	3g.	cinnamon bark	3g.
astragalus	2.5-3g.	white peony	3g.	licorice	1.5g.
ovate atractylodes	3g.	rehmannia	3g.		
poria	3g.	ligusticum	3g.		

PATTERN

Constitutional state   5 4 3 (2 1)

Signs and symptoms

Asthenia .... • <u>easy fatigability, lack of strength, debilitated state</u>
• spontaneous sweating, night sweating
• poor appetite
• cold extremities, chills

Blood imbalance .... • <u>signs of blood vacuity</u>
• chronic bleeding

TCM pattern identification

Qi-blood dual vacuity

APPLICATIONS

Abnormal bleeding/menstrual disorders/vaginal symptoms ....
• dysfunctional uterine bleeding, menstrual disorders and abnormal vaginal discharge associated with chronic debilitating disorders, atrophic vaginitis

Urinary disorders .... • may be beneficial in incontinence

Osteoporosis .... • may be beneficial in osteoporosis

ADDITIONAL APPLICATIONS

Chronic hepatitis, ulcerative colitis, anemic conditions, postpartum care, poor wound healing, malignancies

NOTES

This formula is indicated for insufficiency of both the functional and material aspects of the body, generally associated with chronic disorders.

Useful in recovery from debilitating disorders or surgery (promotes proper healing of wounds). Beneficial as an adjunct in anticancer drug or radiation therapy (helps to counter adverse side effects such as leucopenia, anemia, anorexia, etc.)

See Prevention of GI disturbances, p. 85.

Substances on the Caution List: cinnamon, ginseng, licorice, ligusticum, peony, *rehmannia, tangkuei.

Contraindications

Except for chronic recurrent low grade fever (such as seen in consumptive disorders) or heat in the palms and soles, do not prescribe in fever/heat is present.

Not suitable for severely debilitated conditions.

PINELLIA AND MAGNOLIA BARK DECOCTION
Hangekōbokutō   *bàn xià hòu pò tāng*

COMPOSITION

processed pinellia	5-6g.	perilla leaf	2g.
poria	5g.	fresh ginger	3-4g.
magnolia bark	3g.		

PATTERN

Constitutional state   5 (4 3 2) 1

Typical traits/predisposing factors
Nervous temperament

Signs and symptoms
<u>Sensation of a lump in the throat</u>, or any discomfort in the throat area felt to interfere with breathing or swallowing. Associated with upper abdominal discomfort or bloating or substernal splashing sound. Usually occurs in attacks.

Fluid stagnation .... • GI disturbances such as substernal discomfort or bloating, eructation, poor appetite, nausea, vomiting
- tendency to edema
- sputum (associated with coughing or dyspnea)

Others .... • psychologic symptoms such as anxiety, depressed mood, insomnia, palpitations (or throbbing felt in the neck, head, hand or other parts of the body)

Abdominal findings .... • substernal splashing sound
- substernal hard glomus
- periumbilical pulsation

TCM pattern identification
Plum-pit qi (phlegm-qi bind), counterflow ascent of stomach qi associated with phlegm-rheum, lung qi counterflow associated with phlegm-damp

APPLICATIONS

Emotional distress .... • anxiety, depression, neurotic conditions featuring globus hystericus

Abnormal bleeding/menstrual disorders/vaginal symptoms ....
- can be applied in menstrual disorders related to psychological stress

Urinary disorders .... • may be useful as an adjunct in nervous frequent urination or other urinary disorders with a strong psychogenic factor

ADDITIONAL APPLICATIONS

Irritation, swelling, pain or itching in the throat area, as in: ....
- tonsillitis, bronchitis, coughing, hyperthyroidism, asthma, spasm of the esophagus, pharyngitis, lump in the throat sensation after upper abdominal surgery

GI .... • gastritis, hyperacidity, gastric atony, nervous vomiting, vomiting in pregnancy

NOTES

This formula should not be prescribed automatically for lump in the throat sensation. Other formulas that may also ameliorate the condition include:

Counterflow Cold Powder

Bupleurum, Cinnamon Twig and Dried Ginger Decoction

Bupleurum Decoction Plus Dragon Bone and Oyster Shell

Supplemented Free Wanderer Powder

Cinnamon Twig Decoction Plus Dragon Bone and Oyster Shell

Poria, Cinnamon Twig, Ovate Atractylodes and Licorice Decoction

Cyperus and Perilla Powder

Combination with a bupleurum formula may be appropriate.

Substances on the Caution List: ginger, magnolia bark, perilla leaf, pinellia.

Contraindications: Due to the drying effect of this formula, administration is not advised in cases without any of the above indication of fluid stagnation (including substernal splashing sound). Discontinue use if the tongue begins to appear dry. Do not prescribe for anemic or weak individuals with marked soft and weak abdomen.

PINELLIA HEART-DRAINING DECOCTION

Hangeshashintō   *bàn xià xiè xīn tāng*

COMPOSITION

pinellia	4-5g.	ginseng	2.5-3g.	coptis	1g.
scutellaria	2.5-3g.	licorice	2.5-3g.		
dried ginger	2-2.5g.	jujube	2.5-3g.		

PATTERN

Constitutional state   5 (4 3 2) 1

Signs and symptoms

GI disturbances .... • substernal discomfort

• abdominal rumbling

• nausea, vomiting

• mild diarrhea or tendency to diarrhea

• poor appetite

Others .... •neck and shoulder stiffness

Abdominal findings .... •substernal hard glomus

• substernal splashing sound

TC pattern identification

Spleen-stomach disharmony

APPLICATIONS

Emotional distress............. • nervous indigestion, nausea and vomiting or diarrhea; gastrointestinal neurosis (such as aerophagia); other neurotic conditions with GI symptoms

Body aches and pain, osteoporosis ....

• normalizes the digestive function and enhances calcium absorption; may be beneficial in osteoporosis

ADDITIONAL APPLICATIONS

GI .... • dyspepsia, gastritis, gastric atony, peptic ulcer, iatrogenic gastric problems, enteritis, irritable bowel syndrome, stomatitis

Others .... •vomiting in pregnancy, motion sickness, hangover

NOTES

Frequently prescribed for upper alimentary tract disorders.

Raw ginger may be added for frequent belching and heartburn, or offensive-smelling flatus.

Use Licorice Heart-Draining Decoction (Pinellia Heart-Draining Decoction with increased amount of licorice) if diarrhea is frequent or severe; or if pain or psychologic symptoms (such as restlessness, insomnia, and mood swings) are more acute. Licorice Heart-Draining Decoction may also be applied in various sleep disturbances, including difficulty in initiating or maintaining sleep, non-restorative sleep, dream-troubled sleep, talking in sleep, and somnambulism.

Substances on the Caution List: coptis, ginger, ginseng, jujube, *licorice, pinellia.

PINELLIA, OVATE ATRACTYLODES AND GASTRODIA DECOCTION
Hangebyakujutsutenmatō   bàn xià bái zhú tiān má tāng

COMPOSITION

processed pinellia	3g.	ginseng	1.5g.	phellodendron	1.5g.
ovate atractylodes	3-6g.	alisma	1.5g.	fresh ginger	0.5-2g.
red tangerine peel	3g.	gastrodia	2g.	dried ginger	0.5-1g.
poria	3g.	barley sprout	1.5-2g.		
astragalus	1.5g	medicated leaven	2g.		

PATTERN

Constitutional state   5 4 (3 2 1)

Signs and symptoms

Fluid imbalance .... • <u>dizziness</u>, ranging from slight giddiness to rocking, floating, or up-side-down sensation; or vertigo
• heavy-headedness (or bag-over-the-head sensation), sensation of pressure in the head
• headache
• nausea, vomiting, or retching
• palpitations

Asthenia .... • <u>weak digestive function</u>
• pale complexion
• easy fatigability
• cold extremities

Abdominal findings .... • substernal splashing sound
• substernal hard glomus

TCM pattern identification
Spleen-stomach qi vacuity, phlegm turbidity harassing the upper body, phlegm inversion headache

APPLICATIONS

Chronic headaches .... • applicable in tension headaches, headaches associated with heavy-headedness or dizziness; can be effective for headaches associated with hypertension
• acute symptoms often triggered by incipient bad weather; can also be brought on by emotional stress, dietary indiscretion, or other adverse stimuli

Hypertension .... • applicable in abnormal blood pressure (high or low)

ADDITIONAL APPLICATIONS

Meniere's disease, chronic dizziness, gastric atony, chronic gastroenteritis, cerebrovascular disease

NOTE

Substances on the Caution List: ginger, ginseng, pinellia.

POLYPORUS DECOCTION

Choreitō   *zhū líng tāng*

COMPOSITION					
polyporus	3g.	talcum	3g.	ass hide glue	3g.
poria	3g.	alisma	3g.		

PATTERN

Constitutional state   5 (4 3 2) 1

Signs and symptoms

Fluid imbalance .... • <u>urinary symptoms</u>–dysuria, frequency, sense of incomplete voiding, concentrated urine, cloudy urine, hematuria

• edema or sense of heaviness below the waist

• diarrhea

Heat .... • thirst

• inflammation (urinary tract, lower alimentary tract)

• heat sensations

• restlessness, insomnia

Abdominal findings .... • lower abdomen may be tense or tender to pressure

TCM pattern identification

Binding of water and heat, with features of yin vacuity

APPLICATIONS

Urinary disorders .... • cystourethritis (mild inflammation), urethral syndrome and other urinary problems not explained by urologic findings, incontinence

ADDITIONAL APPLICATIONS

Urinary .... • nephritis, nephrosis, urinary calculi, pyelitis, renal tuberculosis

GI .... • diarrhea, enteritis

NOTES

In urinary disorders with more evidence of inflammation, consider Gentian Liver-Draining Decoction or Five Stranguries Powder. However, this formula is more effective for hematuria.

In recurrent or chronic cases with signs of blood vacuity and in the absence of digestive disorders, prescribe Polyporus Decoction Combined with Four Agents Decoction. (For this combination of formulas, Substances on the Caution List are ligusticum, peony, *rehmannia, and tangkuei.)

PORIA, CINNAMON TWIG, OVATE ATRACTYLODES AND LICORICE DECOCTION

Ryōkeijutsukantō   *líng guì zhú gān tāng*

COMPOSITION

poria	6g.	ovate atractylodes	3g.
cinnamon twig	4g.	honey-fried licorice	2g.

PATTERN

Constitutional state   5 (4 3 2) 1

Typical traits/predisposing factors

Gastric atony; hypotension

Signs and symptoms

Fluid imbalance .... • <u>dizziness</u> (all types, including dizziness when rising or changing positions and vertigo)
  • palpitations
  • shortness of breath
  • substernal discomfort
  • headaches
  • reduced urinary output (without thirst) or nervous frequent urination
  • tinnitus
  • twitching or pulsation felt in the face, arms or other parts of the body

Others .... • headrushes

Abdominal findings .... • substernal splashing sound or substernal hard glomus
  • periumbilical pulsation
  • mild upper rectus tension

TCM pattern identification

Phlegm-rheum associated with spleen vacuity, water damp with cold signs

APPLICATIONS

Hot flushes and other vasomotor manifestations

Emotional distress .... • may be beneficial in conditions characterized by dizziness and palpitations

Chronic headaches

ADDITIONAL APPLICATIONS

Postural hypotension, Meniere's disease, myopia spuria, heart diseases, motion sickness

NOTES

Substances on the Caution List: cinnamon, licorice.

PORIA FIVE POWDER

Goreisan   *wŭ líng săn*

COMPOSITION

alisma	5-6g.	poria	3-4.5g.	cinnamon twig	2-3g.
polyporus	3-4.5g.	ovate atractylodes	3-4.5g.		

PATTERN

Constitutional state   5 (4 3 2) 1

Signs and symptoms

Fluid imbalance .... • <u>thirst</u> despite intake of fluids, or immediate ejection of ingested fluids

• <u>reduced urinary output</u>

• edema, or a sense of heaviness

• vomiting

• diarrhea

• dizziness

• substernal discomfort

Others .... • headache

Abdominal findings .... • substernal splashing sound, or borborygmi when the substernal region is pressed

• periumbilical pulsation

• substernal hard glomus

TCM pattern identification

Water damp, exterior pattern with water damp, water counterflow

APPLICATIONS

Chronic headaches .... • headaches without special characteristics may respond to this remedy, but it is most effective for attacks of migraines and other headaches that are preceded or accompanied by the symptoms of fluid imbalance specified above

Urinary disorders .... • may be useful in cystourethritis, urethral syndrome, and other disorders not explained by urologic findings

• may be beneficial in incontinence if the characteristic symptoms are present

ADDITIONAL APPLICATIONS	
Urinary	• nephritis, nephrotic syndrome, uremia
GI	• dyspepsia, gastric dilatation, gastroptosis, gastritis, enteritis
Hormonal-metabolic	• diabetes mellitus
EENT	• myopia spuria, chronic conjunctivitis, Meniere's disease
Nervous	• epilepsy, trigeminal neuralgia
Others	• common cold, heat exhaustion, vomiting in pregnancy, hangover

NOTES

To be taken with cold water when there is nausea or vomiting.

Originally intended as a powder, but the decoction form is also employed traditionally. The powder format is considered by some to be more efficacious. Its daily dosage is as follows:

polyporus	1.1g.	poria	1.1g.
alisma	1.9g.	cinnamon	0.8g.
ovate atractylodes	1.1g.		

for a total of 6.0g., to be taken in 3 divided doses. 1-2g. of the powder may be taken on an as-needed basis for acute conditions.

When fluid ingested is immediately vomited, it is necessary to use the powder format. Dissolve it in cold rice water and take a little at a time. The rice water, or thin rice gruel, may be made by mixing powdered rice with hot water.

Substances on the Caution List: cinnamon.

PORIA, GINGER, OVATE ATRACTYLODES AND LICORICE DECOCTION
Ryōkyōjutsukantō   *líng jiāng zhú gān tāng*

COMPOSITION

poria	6g.	ovate atractylodes	3g.
dried ginger	3g.	licorice	2g.

PATTERN

Constitutional state   5 4 (3 2 1)

Signs and symptoms

Coldness syndrome .... • coldness in the lumbar region or from the lumbar region downward, with attendant pain or sense of heaviness

• symptoms aggravated by exposure to cold and dampness

Fluid imbalance .... • frequent urination or long micturition without unusual thirst

• edema

TCM pattern identification

Cold damp in the lower burner

APPLICATION

Abnormal bleeding/menstrual disorders/vaginal symptoms ....

• may be beneficial in abnormal vaginal discharge, atrophic vaginitis, menstrual disorders

Urinary disorders .... • chronic cystourethritis, urethral syndrome and other disorders not explained by urologic findings, frequent urination, polyuria, nocturia, incontinence

Body aches and pains, osteoporosis ....

• low back pain, sciatica

• may be beneficial in osteoporosis

ADDITIONAL APPLICATIONS

Gestational nephropathy, eczema in the genital area and lower extremities

NOTE

Substances on the Caution List: ginger, licorice.

Contraindications: Ginger may exacerbate inflammation of the urinary tract. Although this risk is moderated by the demulcent action of licorice, avoid the use of this formula in cases with evident irritative symptoms.

PUERARIA DECOCTION

Kakkontō   *gé gēn tāng*

COMPOSITION

pueraria	4-8g.	cinnamon twig	2-3g.	dried ginger	1g.
ephedra	3-4g.	white peony	2-3g.		
jujube	3-4g.	licorice	2g.		

PATTERN

Constitutional state   (5 4) 3 2 1

Signs and symptoms

Marked tightness and stiffness of the muscles in the neck and/or back in acute stage of painful conditions (see note below)

Others .... • associated symptoms vary; consult "Additional Applications"

Abdominal findings .... • may have supraumbilical tenderness

TCM pattern identification

Exterior cold, exterior repletion

APPLICATIONS

Chronic headaches .... • acute headaches with stiff neck (and back); migraines; headaches associated with chronic problems of the nose or paranasal sinuses (more effective with the addition of ligusticum and magnolia flower, i.e., Pueraria Decoction Plus Ligusticum and Magnolia)

Body aches and pains .... • stiffness and pain in the neck, shoulders or back; fibrositis

ADDITIONAL APPLICATIONS

Febrile disorders (initial stage, with marked chill) ....
                            • influenza, common cold, acute colitis, acute tonsillitis, bronchitis, measles, viral menigitis

Inflammatory/suppurative conditions in the head or upper body (generally require addition of other substances) ....
                            • conjunctivitis, otitis media, sinusitis, rhinitis, gingivitis, furuncle, lymphadenopathy, mastitis

Others .... • neuralgia (trigeminal, intercostal), insufficient milk production

NOTES

This formula is suitable for muscular tightness that extends longitudinally from the neck to the back (compare muscular tightness treated with bupleurum formulas, which extends laterally from shoulder to shoulder). Also, fluid congestion is generally evident. Check for this by gently pinching the skin in a section of the affected region. The skin will feel thick, and the maneuver may be painful for the patient. This subcuteneous edema is often associated with pathological changes in the ear, nose, throat, or back of the head.

Pueraria Decoction Plus Atractylodes and Aconite may be prescribed for pain exacerbated by coldness, with evidence of edema (such as swollen joint) or oliguria.

See note on ephedra in Appendix A. May provoke a temporary worsening of symptoms. To minimize the possibility of adverse effects from misuse of this formula, start with a small dose or have the patient take it after eating.

Substances on the Caution List: cinnamon, *ephedra, ginger, jujube, licorice, peony.

Contraindication: spontaneous sweating or tendency to spontaneous sweating.

STRING OF PEARLS BEVERAGE

Renjuin   *lián zhū yǐn*

COMPOSITION

poria	5g.	licorice	2g.	white peony	3g.
cinnamon twig	3-4g.	tangkuei	3g.	rehmannia	3g.
ovate atractylodes	3g.	ligusticum	3g.		

PATTERN

Constitutional state   5 4 (3 2) 1

Signs and symptoms

Blood vacuity and fluid imbalance ....

- <u>palpitations</u>
- <u>dizziness, dizziness when rising or changing position</u>
- mild edema in the face or lower limbs, or mild constitutional edema
- tinnitus
- shortness of breath
- flushing and profuse sweating
- headache
- other indications of blood vacuity

Abdominal findings ....
- soft wall with periumbilical pulsations
- substernal splashing sound

TCM pattern identification

Blood vacuity with water damp

APPLICATIONS

Hot flushes and other vasomotor manifestations ....
- applicable in severe hot flushes

ADDITIONAL APPLICATIONS

Mild anemic conditions associated with pregnancy, hemorrhoidal bleeding, heart diseases, etc.

NOTES

This remedy is derived from the combination of Poria, Cinnamon Twig, Ovate Atractylodes and Licorice Decoction with Four Agents Decoction.

See Prevention of GI Disturbances, p. 85.

Substances on the Caution List: cinnamon, licorice, ligusticum, peony, *rehmannia, tangkuei.

RHUBARB AND MOUTAN DECOCTION
Daiōbotanpitō   *dà huáng mǔ dān pí tāng*

COMPOSITION

rhubarb	1-2g.	peach kernel	4g.	wax gourd seed	4-6g.
moutan	4g.	mirabilite	4g.		

PATTERN

Constitutional state   (5 4) 3 2 1

Signs and symptoms

Blood stasis .... • pelvic congestion syndrome
                                   • menstrual disorders
                                   • other local or general indications of blood stasis

Heat .... • inflammation in the lower body

Others .... • tendency to constipation

Abdominal findings .... • <u>blood stasis signs</u>, esp. in the RLQ

TCM pattern identification

Blood stasis with interior repletion heat, yong of the intestine

APPLICATIONS

Hot flushes and other vasomotor manifestations

Abnormal bleeding/menstrual disorders/vaginal symptoms ....
                                   • dysfunctional uterine bleeding, dysmenorrhea, irregular menstruation, PMS, vaginitis

Urinary disorders .... • cystourethritis (esp. when urinary obstruction accompanies acute inflammation), urethral syndrome and other disorders not explained by urologic findings

ADDITIONAL APPLICATIONS

Gynecologic .... • pelvic inflammatory disease, endometriosis, bartholinitis, infertility, prolapse of uterus

GI .... • initial stage of appendicitis (prior to suppuration), ulcerative colitis, enteritis, Crohn's disease, proctitis, constipation, hemorrhoids

Urogenital .... • urinary calculi, pyelitis, gonorrhea

NOTE

Substances on the Caution List: *mirabilite, moutan, peach kernel, *rhubarb.

SEVEN AGENTS DOWNBEARING DECOCTION
Shichimotsukōkatō   *qī wù jiàng xià tāng*

<table>
<tr><td colspan="6">COMPOSITION</td></tr>
<tr><td>tangkuei</td><td>3-4g.</td><td>rehmannia</td><td>3-4g.</td><td>phellodendron</td><td>2g.</td></tr>
<tr><td>peony</td><td>3-4g.</td><td>uncaria</td><td>3-4g.</td><td></td><td></td></tr>
<tr><td>ligusticum</td><td>3-4g.</td><td>astragalus</td><td>2-3g.</td><td></td><td></td></tr>
</table>

PATTERN

Constitutional state   5 4 (3 2) 1

Signs and symptoms

Headrush syndrome .... • associated symptoms include headaches, dizziness, heavy-headedness, shoulder stiffness, tinnitus, ocular rubor (or retinal hemorrhage)

Blood vacuity .... • dry lusterless skin
 • tingling or numbness in the extremities
 • muscle spasms

Others .... • easy fatigability
 • cold extremities

Abdominal findings .... • soft abdomen with periumbilical pulsation

TCM pattern identification

Blood vacuity and liver yang transforming into wind

APPLICATIONS

Hot flushes and other vasomotor manifestations

Chronic headaches .... • tension headaches, migraines

Hypertension, hyperlipidemia, atherosclerosis ....
 • may also be applicable in hypertension associated with kidney disorders

ADDITIONAL APPLICATIONS

Stroke (hemiplegia), chronic nephritis, nephrotic syndrome

NOTE

See Prevention of GI Disturbances, p. 85.

Substances on the Caution List: ligusticum, peony, *rehmannia, tangkuei.

Contraindication: Not suitable for persons having marked weakness of the digestive function.

SIX GENTLEMEN DECOCTION

Rikkunshitō   *liù jūn zǐ tāng*

COMPOSITION

ginseng	2-4g.	pinellia	3-4g.	fresh ginger	1-2g.
ovate atractylodes	3-4g.	tangerine peel	2-4g.	jujube	2g.
poria	3-4g.	licorice	1-1.5g.		

PATTERN

Constitutional state   5 4 (3 2) 1

Signs and symptoms

Asthenia .... • <u>fatigue, easy fatigability</u>, lack of strength
• lusterless complexion
• cold extremities

Weak digestive function ..... • <u>poor appetite</u>
• <u>substernal discomfort</u>
• eructations, abdominal rumbling
• sluggishness or drowsiness after eating
• tendency to diarrhea or atonic constipation
• nausea, vomiting

Others .... • stiff shoulders

Abdominal findings .... • <u>substernal splashing sound</u>
• substernal hard glomus(or hypotonicity)
• hypotonic lower abdomen

TCM pattern identification

Spleen-stomach qi vacuity with phlegm-damp,
qi vacuity with stagnation of qi or water

APPLICATIONS

Body aches and pains, osteoporosis ....
• may be beneficial for shoulder stiffness associated with weak digestive function
• may be useful in osteoporosis (normalizes the GI function, promotes the absorption of calcium)

ADDITIONAL APPLICATIONS

GI .... • chronic indigestion, chronic gastritis, gastric atony, peptic ulcer

NOTES

Broadly applicable for the purpose of improving the digestive function or reducing the GI side effects of drugs.

Substances on the Caution List: ginger, ginseng, jujube, licorice, pinellia.

SPINY JUJUBE DECOCTION

Sansōnintō   *suān zǎo rén tāng*

COMPOSITION					
spiny jujube	7-15g.	ligusticum	3g.	licorice	1g.
anemarrhena	3g.	poria	5g.		

PATTERN

Constitutional state   5 (4 3 2) 1

Signs and symptoms

Asthenia ....• exhausted or debilitated state

• night sweating

Psychologic symptoms .... • poor sleep (typically associated with vexation) or hypersomnia

Others ....• dizziness

TCM pattern identification

Heart blood vacuity with heat signs

APPLICATIONS

Sleep disturbances .... • difficulty in maintaining sleep, nonrestorative sleep, dream-troubled sleep, excessive sleepiness

NOTES

This formula is beneficial in cases of poor sleep where the person does not sleep deeply, awakes often and has many dreams. It is particularly suitable for poor sleep occurring with utter exhaustion.

May be employed adjunctively alongside other remedies for insomnia characterized by difficulty in initiating sleep. Dosage should be adjusted to individual need.

Use cautiously in patients with weak digestive function. See Prevention of GI Disturbances, p. 85.

Substances on the Caution List: spiny jujube kernel, licorice, ligusticum.

SPLEEN-EFFUSING DECOCTION PLUS OVATE ATRACTYLODES
Eppikajutsutō   *yuè bì jiā zhú tāng*

COMPOSITION

ephedra	6g.	ovate atractylodes	4g.	jujube	3g.
gypsum	8g.	fresh ginger	3g.	licorice	2g.

PATTERN

Constitutional state   (5 4 3) 2 1

Signs and symptoms

Fluid imbalance.................
- acute stage of local inflammatory edema or acute constitutional edema (indentation made by a finger pressed into skin swollen by edema flattens out quickly)
- decreased urinary output
- tendency to spontaneous perspiration (or broadly, exudation onto the body surface, as in "weeping" skin conditions or excessive tearing of the eyes)

Heat ....
- rubor and heat in the affected area
- thirst or mouth dryness

Abdominal findings............
- possibly, an unusual warmth may be palpable in the center of the chest, and points on the anterior midline over the sternum may be tender to pressure

TCM pattern identification
Wind water or water swelling with heat, heat bi, wind damp-heat

APPLICATIONS

Body aches and pains.........
- arthritis with heat, rubor, and swelling (acute stage or flare-ups)
- may be combined with formulas such as Cinnamon Twig Decoction Plus Atractylodes and Aconite and Fangji and Astragalus Decoction to treat local heat and swelling

ADDITIONAL APPLICATIONS

Nephritis, nephrosis, gout, jaundice, varicose veins, skin problems featuring blisters or much discharge (e.g., atopy, pemphigoid), keloids, pterygium, blepharitis

NOTES

See notes on ephedra and gypsum in Appendix A. To minimize the possibility of adverse effects from misuse of this formula, start with a small dose or have the patient take it after eating.

Substances on the Caution List: *ephedra, ginger, gypsum, jujube, licorice.

SPLEEN-RETURNING DECOCTION

Kihitō   *guī pí tāng*

COMPOSITION

ginseng	2-3g.	licorice	1g.	astragalus	2-3g.
root poria	2-3g.	jujube	1-2g.	polygala	1-2g.
longan flesh	2-3g.	ovate atractylodes	2-3g.	saussurea	1g.
tangkuei	2g.	spiny jujube	2-3g.	dried ginger	1-1.5g.

PATTERN

Constitutional state   5 4 (3 2 1)

Typical traits/predisposing factors

Excessive pondering or worrying

Signs and symptoms

Asthenia ....• <u>fatigue, easy fatigability</u>

• <u>weak digestive function</u>

• short shallow breathing

• night sweating

<u>Psychologic symptoms</u> (associated with fatigue, esp. mental exhaustion) anxiety, depressed mood, insomnia, inability to concentrate, impaired memory, loss of interest

Blood imbalance ....• chronic recurrent bleeding disorders (e.g., subcutaneous or uterine)

• blood vacuity or anemia

Abdominal findings ....• periumbilical pulsation

TCM pattern identification

Spleen qi vacuity and heart blood vacuity, spleen failing to manage the blood (qi failing to contain the blood)

APPLICATIONS

Sleep disturbances...............• difficulty in initiating or maintaining sleep, non-restorative sleep, dream-troubled sleep, daytime drowsiness

Emotional distress...............• anxiety, depression, neurotic conditions

Abnormal bleeding/menstrual disorders/vaginal symptoms ....

• chronic abnormal uterine bleeding, irregular menstruation

ADDITIONAL APPLICATIONS	

Blood.................................. • chronic bleeding, hypo-albuminemia, anemic conditions (e.g., leukemia, aplastic anemia, Banti's disease, idiopathic thrombocytopenia)

GI .... • chronic gastroenteritis, nervous gastritis

Others .... • psychosomatic cardiovascular disease

NOTES	

Suitable in conditions without inflammation or hyperemia.

Supplemented Spleen-Returning Decoction (Spleen-Returning Decoction with the addition of bupleurum and gardenia fruit) is applicable when heat symptoms such as headrushes, irritability or slight subcostal distress are present in addition to the above. However, it is generally unsuitable in cases with marked agitation.

TCM pattern identification: above pattern with signs of liver fire

Substances on the Caution List: ginger, ginseng, jujube, licorice, spiny jujube kernel, tangkuei (and gardenia in the supplemented formula).

SUPPLEMENTED FREE WANDERER POWDER
Kamishōyōsan   *jiā wèi xiāo yáo sǎn*

COMPOSITION

tangkuei	3g.	dried ginger	1g.	licorice	1.5-2g.
ovate atractylodes	3g.	white peony	3g.	mint leaf	1g.
bupleurum	3g.	poria	3g.		
gardenia	2g.	moutan	2g.		

PATTERN

Constitutional state   5 4 (3 2) 1

Typical traits/predisposing factors

Nervous temperament

A history of lower abdominal surgery or artificial abortion

Signs and symptoms

Various nonspecific somatic and psychological symptoms (often multiple fluctuating complaints), typically involving the following:

Psychological symptoms ..... • mood swings, tension, irritability, outbursts of pent-up anger, insomnia

Blood imbalance .... • menstrual disorders

Vasomotor symptoms .... • headrushes/hot flushes, chills, sweating, cold extremities, heat in the palms or soles, palpitations, paresthesia, dizziness, headaches

Others .... • easy fatigability, slow recovery from fatigue

• body aches and pains

• diarrhea or difficult bowel movement (thin/pellet-like stool, sense of incomplete evacuation, constipation)

• poor appetite

Abdominal findings .... • slight subcostal distress

• mild blood stasis signs

TCM pattern identification

Depressed liver qi transforming into fire, liver-spleen disharmony; with features of qi-blood dual vacuity

APPLICATIONS

Hot flushes and other vasomotor manifestations

Sleep disturbances .... • difficulty in initiating or maintaining sleep, non restorative sleep, dream-troubled sleep

Emotional distress .... • depression, anxiety, neurotic conditions, nervous problems following gynecologic surgery

Chronic headaches .... • tension headaches, headaches associated with menstrual problems, headaches accompanied by many nonspecific symptoms

Abnormal bleeding/menstrual disorders/vaginal symptoms ....
• dysfunctional uterine bleeding, dysmenorrhea, irregular menstruation, PMS, abnormal vaginal discharge, atrophic vaginitis, vaginitis

Urinary disorders .... • recurrent cystourethritis, urethral syndrome and other disorders unexplained by urologic findings

Body aches and pains .... • fibrositis; stiffness or pain in the neck, shoulder or arm

Hypertension, atherosclerosis ....
• applicable in psychosomatic cardiovascular disease; frequently suitable for hypertension in the perimenopause

ADDITIONAL APPLICATIONS

Gynecologic .... • amenorrhea, infertility, insufficient lactation, pelvic inflammatory disease

Hepato-biliary .... • chronic liver disorders (relatively mild cases of hepatitis B, NANB; incipient cirrhosis)

Others .... • irritable bowel syndrome, hyperthyroidism

NOTES

Widely prescribed for problems in the perimenopause.

Substances on the Caution List: gardenia, ginger, licorice, moutan, peony, tangkuei.

TANGKUEI AND PEONY POWDER
Tōkishakuyakusan   *dāng guī sháo yào sǎn*

COMPOSITION

tangkuei	3g.	peony	4-6g.	ovate atractylodes	4g.
ligusticum	3g.	poria	4g.	alisma	4-5g.

PATTERN

Constitutional state   5 4 (3 2 1)

Signs and symptoms

Asthenia ....
- coldness syndrome (cold lower body and extremities)
- easy fatigability, tired appearance

Fluid imbalance ....
- slack skin (that suggests subcutaneous fluid stagnation), especially under the eyes
- tendency to edema (esp. premenstrual)
- symptoms arising from localized edema such as heavy-headedness, dizziness, headache, tinnitus
- urinary frequency
- palpitations

Blood imbalance ....
- menstrual disorders
- indications of blood vacuity

Others ....
- aches and pains – abdominal pain (gynecologic cause), shoulder stiffness, low back pain, etc.

Abdominal findings ....
- blood stasis signs near the umbilicus
- substernal splashing sound

TCM pattern identification

Blood vacuity and water-damp with signs of blood stasis, spleen vacuity and cold

APPLICATIONS

Hot flushes and other vasomotor manifestations

Emotional distress ....
- mild emotional symptoms associated with blood imbalance

Chronic headaches ....
- tension headaches, headaches associated with gynecologic disorders, headaches associated with hypertension

Abnormal bleeding/menstrual disorders/vaginal symptoms ....
- dysfunctional uterine bleeding, dysmenorrhea, irregular menstruation, PMS; abnormal vaginal discharge, vaginal irritation, atrophic vaginitis (little evidence of inflammation)

Urinary disorders .... • recurrent cystourethritis, urethral syndrome

Body aches and pains, osteoporosis ....

• low back pain, sciatica, fibrositis

• may be beneficial in osteoporosis

Hypertension, hyperlipidemia, atherosclerosis ....

• applicable in both high and low blood pressure

ADDITIONAL APPLICATIONS

Gynecologic .... • amenorrhea, infertility, habitual abortion, toxemia of pregnancy, abdominal pain during pregnancy, pelvic congestion syndrome

Skin .... • acne, chilblains, chloasma, eczema

Urinary .... • chronic nephritis, chronic nephrosis

Other .... • edema, hemorrhoids, Meniere's disease, hypothyroidism

NOTES

Widely applicable in disorders associated with menstruation, pregnancy, childbirth and menopause.

See Prevention of GI Disturbances, p. 85. If so desired, this formula may be taken with a little alcohol to aid the digestion and assimilation of the herbs and augment its efficacy.

The original powder format is less likely to cause GI problems. It is also preferable in cases with atonic constipation, since peony root (present in greater proportion in the powder) contains fibers that act as a bulk laxative and temper its astringent effect. With the extract preparation of the decoction, the addition of rhubarb may be necessary. The daily dosage of the powder format is as follows:

tangkuei	0.4g.
peony	2.2g.
poria	0.6g.
alisma	1.1g.
ligusticum	1.1g.
ovate atractylodes	0.6g.

For chronic conditions (or as a constitutional alterative), Ginseng, Tangkuei and Peony Powder may be preferable, a milder and more tonifying remedy derived from Tangkuei and Peony Powder by reducing the amount of ligusticum (which is often the cause of minor gastric distress) by half and adding ginseng, cinnamon and licorice.

Substances on the Caution List: ligusticum, peony, tangkuei.

TANGKUEI COUNTERFLOW COLD DECOCTION PLUS EVODIA AND FRESH GINGER
Tōkishigyakukagoshuyushōkyōtō
dāng guī sì nì jiā wú zhū yú shēng jiāng tāng

COMPOSITION

tangkuei	3g.	mutong	3g.	jujube	5g.
cinnamon twig	3g.	asarum	2g.	evodia	1-2g.
peony	3g.	licorice	2g.	fresh ginger	4g.

PATTERN

Constitutional state   5 4 (3 2) 1

Typical traits/predisposing factors

Insufficient peripheral circulation

Poor vasomotor adjustment to temperature fluctuations (facial flushing when exposed to warmth; marked cold extremities when exposed to cold)

Symptoms tend to be precipitated or worsened by exposure to cold, including excessive cold food in the diet

Signs and symptoms

Coldness syndrome .... • chronic or severe cold extremities, esp. lower extremities (in severe cases, sufferer may wear socks to bed even in warm weather)
- cold lower body
- pain associated with coldness – especially in the lower abdomen, but also in the back, extremities or head
- paresthesia
- tendency to chilblains

GI disturbances (associated with coldness) ....
- abdominal pain
- nausea, vomiting
- diarrhea

Abdominal findings .... • possibly general rectus tension, or gaseous distention, or tenderness in the lower abdomen

TCM pattern identification

Contract cold in blood vacuity, cold stagnating in the liver vessel, enduring interior cold

APPLICATIONS

Chronic headaches .... • attacks of migraines and other headaches

Abnormal bleeding/menstrual disorders/vaginal symptoms ....
        • may be beneficial in dysmenorrhea, irregular menstruation, abnormal vaginal discharge and atrophic vaginitis

Body aches and pains, osteoporosis ....
        • low back pain, sciatica, fibrositis
        • may be beneficial in osteoporosis

ADDITIONAL APPLICATIONS

Nervous .... • neuralgia, Bell's palsy

CV .... • chilblains, Raynaud's disease, skin disorders with cyanosis, intermittent claudication

Others .... • chronic appendicitis, pelvic peritonitis, colic, peptic ulcer, functional disturbances from exposure to cold, hand eczema, hypothyroidism

NOTES

Improves the circulation and warms up the body. Can be taken from autumn to winter as a prophylactic and treatment for chilblains or frostbite.

Very bitter-tasting, but the taste tends to be well tolerated by patients with the above pattern.

More effective when taken with a little alcohol (originally decocted with equal volumes of water and wine).

For less chronic cases or cases without nausea/vomiting and headaches, Tangkuei Counterflow Cold Decoction without the addition of evodia and ginger may be suitable.

Substances on the Caution List: cinnamon, evodia, ginger, jujube, licorice, mutong, peony, tangkuei.

TEN-INGREDIENT TOXIN-VANQUISHING DECOCTION
Jūmihaidokutō   *shí wèi bài dú tāng*

COMPOSITION

bupleurum	2-3g.	poria	2-4g.	fresh ginger	1-3g.
cherry bark	2-3g.	tuhuo	1.5-3g.	schizonepeta	1-1.5g.
platycodon	2-3g.	ledebouriella	1.5-3g.	forsythia	0/2-3g.
ligusticum	2-3g.	licorice	1-1.5g.		

(None or up to 2-3g. of forsythia may be used.)

PATTERN

Constitutional state   5 (4 3 2) 1

Typical traits/predisposing factors

Tendency to pyoderma; atopy

Signs and symptoms

<u>Initial stage of suppurative skin conditions, or allergic dermatitis</u> (little or no discharge)

Abdominal findings .... • subcostal distress

TCM pattern identification

Wind-damp-heat skin eruptions

APPLICATIONS

Abnormal bleeding/menstrual disorders/vaginal symptoms ....
- may be applied when there is mild to moderate degree of rubor, swelling and itching of the external genitals, such as in atrophic vaginitis, vaginitis and incipient suppurative conditions in the external genitals

ADDITIONAL APPLICATIONS

Skin .... • eczema, dermatitis, acne, urticaria, boils, furuncle, carbuncle

EENT .... • allergic ophthalmia, sty, otitis externa, otitis media, sinusitis

Others .... • lymphadenopathy, mastitis

NOTES

Originally created to treat the initial stage of suppurative skin disorders, Ten-Ingredient Toxin-Vanquishing Decoction can also be beneficial in a variety of allergic skin problems. Certain practitioners also consider it to be a constitutional alterative for these conditions.

The constitutional state is of little concern in its application. However, it can be particularly useful for individuals with various allergies, food or drug sensitivities. For this reason, this formula is included as a potential remedy in the treatment of vulvovaginitis although it is not commonly employed in this regard.

Depending on the maker, the extract may or may not be formulated with forsythia. Its inclusion is desirable if there is a tendency to suppuration.

May possibly provoke a temporary worsening of symptoms.

Substances on the Caution List: ginger, ledebouriella, licorice, ligusticum, schizonepeta.

TRUE WARRIOR DECOCTION
Shinbutō   *zhēn wǔ tāng*

COMPOSITION

ovate atractylodes 3g.	white peony 3g.	processed aconite 0.5-1g.
poria 4-5g.	dried ginger 1.5g.	

PATTERN

Constitutional state   5 4 3 (2 1)

Signs and symptoms

Asthenia .... • lack of vitality (desire to be recumbent), easy fatigability
  • coldness syndrome–cold extremities, general lack of body warmth
  • pallor

Fluid imbalance .... • diarrhea or tendency to diarrhea (typically watery stool followed by feeling of weakness, without thirst)
  • dizziness (ranging from light-headedness on rising to sensation of riding in a moving vehicle to vertigo; may also be dizzy when recumbent)
  • palpitations
  • reduced urinary output
  • sense of heaviness in the limbs
  • pitting edema
  • aches and pains

Abdominal findings .... • substernal splashing sound
  • gaseous distention

TCM pattern identification

Yang vacuity water flood

APPLICATIONS

Chronic headaches

Urinary disorders .... • may be applied in recurrent cystourethritis or incontinence

Body aches and pains .... • may benefit rheumatic conditions with the above pattern

Hypertension .... • applicable in abnormal blood pressure (high or low)

ADDITIONAL APPLICATIONS

GI .... • chronic diarrhea, enteritis, colitis, irritable bowel syndrome

Skin .... • pruritus senilis, urticaria, eczema

Others .... • convalescence from febrile disorders (influenza, bronchitis, pneumonia, etc.), Meniere's disease, nephrotic syndrome, hypothyroidism

NOTE

Substances on the Caution List: *aconite, ginger, peony.

UNCARIA POWDER

Chōtōsan   *gōu téng sǎn*

COMPOSITION

uncaria	3g.	gypsum	5-7g.	ophiopogon	3g.
tangerine peel	3g.	ledebouriella	2g.	poria	3g.
licorice	1g.	chrysanthemum	2g.	ginseng	2g.
dried ginger	1g.	pinellia	3g.		

PATTERN

Constitutional state   5 (4 3 2) 1

Signs and symptoms

Headrush syndrome .... • headrushes (flushing)
  • headache or heavy-headedness
  • dizziness
  • muscular tension in the neck-shoulder area
  • other associated symptoms include ocular rubor, tinnitus, thirst

Psychologic symptoms .... • nervousness, irritability, gloominess, insomnia

Others .... • eye fatigue or pain
  • poor appetite

TCM pattern identification

Liver inversion dizziness, liver yang transforming into wind; with features of spleen qi vacuity and phlegm-damp

APPLICATIONS

Hot flushes and other vasomotor manifestations

Sleep disturbances

Emotional distress .... • depression, neurotic conditions

Chronic headaches .... • especially suitable for headaches or heavy-headedness on waking that subside during the day (often associated with cerebrovascular arteriosclerosis)
  • also useful in general for perimenopausal headaches and dizziness, headaches associated with hypertension, tension headaches, migraines and other vascular headaches

Hypertension, atherosclerosis ....
  • can be of particular benefit in cerebral arteriosclerosis and other cerebrovascular disorders; may be useful in treating aftereffects of stroke

ADDITIONAL APPLICATIONS

Meniere's disease, tinnitus, glaucoma, dementia

NOTES

Substances on the Caution List: ginger, ginseng, gypsum, ledebouriella, licorice, pinellia.

WARM CLEARING BEVERAGE

Unseiin   *wēn qīng yǐn*

COMPOSITION

tangkuei	3-4g.	gardenia	1.5-2g.	scutellaria	1.5-3g.
peony	3-4g.	rehmannia	3-4g.	phellodendron	1.5-2g.
coptis	1.5-2g.	ligusticum	3-4g.		

PATTERN

Constitutional state   5 (4 3 2) 1

Typical traits/predisposing factors

atopy

Signs and symptoms

Blood imbalance .... • dry lusterless skin (mild degree of blood vacuity)
                                • menstrual disorders
                                • bleeding

Heat .... • tendency to headrush syndrome–associated symptoms include flushing, ocular rubor, tinnitus, headache, dizziness, palpitations, thirst
                                • skin problems typically marked by dryness, rubor and itching
                                • hyperemic or inflammatory conditions in general
                                • psychologic symptoms such as anxiety, irritability, restlessness, insomnia

Abdominal findings .... • blood stasis signs

TCM pattern identification

Blood heat (or damp-heat) and blood vacuity

APPLICATIONS

Hot flushes and other vasomotor manifestations

Emotional distress .... • anxiety, depression, neurotic conditions

Abnormal bleeding/menstrual disorders/vaginal symptoms ....
                                • dysfunctional uterine bleeding, dysmenorrhea, irregular menstruation, PMS, vaginitis, atrophic vaginitis

Hypertension, hyperlipidemia, atherosclerosis

ADDITIONAL APPLICATIONS

Gynecologic .... • pelvic inflammatory disease, endometriosis, vicarious menstruation

Skin .... • urticaria, eczema, allergic dermatitis, acne, chloasma, pruritus senilis, rosacea

Bleeding disorders .... • nosebleed, bleeding hemorrhoids, hematemesis, hematuria

Others .... • stomatitis, Behcet's syndrome

NOTES

This is a composite formula made up of Coptis Toxin-Resolving Decoction (a representative formula for heat pattern) and Four Agents Decoction, a basic formula for blood vacuity not introduced in this book. Depending on the needs of the patient, the proportion of the two component formulas may possibly be varied by mixing the respective extracts.

Mainly employed in gynecologic disorders and skin problems.

Very bitter-tasting, but the taste tends to be well tolerated by patients manifesting the above pattern.

Substances on the Caution List: coptis, gardenia, ligusticum, peony, *rehmannia, tangkuei.

Contraindication: Not suitable in persons with marked weak digestive function.

Appendix A: Caution List

This appendix compiles a list of potential adverse effects associated with certain component substances in the context of formula extract therapy.

Consult the table for the type(s) of adverse effects associated with a particular substance, then refer to the corresponding section(s) in the text for more information.[1]

POTENTIAL ADVERSE EFFECTS / SUBSTANCE	I. Allergies, skin symptoms	II. Metabolic disturbances	III. Nervous system effects	IV. GI disturbances	V. Use with caution/avoid in excessive menstrual bleeding & pregnancy
Achyranthes					●
Aconite			●		
Carthamus					●
Cinnamon	●				●
Coix					●
Coptis				●	
Corydalis					●
Ephedra	●		●		
Evodia					●
Gardenia				●	
Ginger	●			●	●
Ginseng	●	●			
Gypsum				●	
Jujube	●				
Ledebouriella	●				
Licorice		●			
Ligusticum	●			●	●
Magnolia (bark, flower)					●
Mirabilite				●	●
Moutan					●
Mutong					●
Notopterygium	●				
Peach kernel				●	●
Peony	●				
Perilla leaf	●				
Pinellia					●
Rehmannia				●	
Rhubarb				●	●
Sappan					●
Schizonepeta	●				
Spiny jujube kernel				●	●
Tangkuei	●			●	
Unripe bitter orange					●

[1] More complete information may be found in, for example, Chinese Herbal Medicine: Materia Medica (see Bibliography).

I. Allergies, skin symptoms

The following substances may worsen existing skin conditions, or cause rashes/itching or other allergic reactions in susceptible patients.[2]

Cinnamon
Ephedra
Ginger (Use cautiously in inflammations of the urinary tract.)
Ginseng
Jujube
Ledebouriella
Ligusticum
Notopterygium
Peony
Perilla leaf
Schizonepeta
Tangkuei

II. Metabolic disturbances

Ginseng

Unlike custom in the West, ginseng is hardly ever employed alone in Kampo. The one exception is Ginseng Solo Decoction, given following acute hemorrhage. Hypertension, insomnia, palpitations, headaches – side effects associated with the overuse of ginseng that are publicized in the US – are unlikely when it is taken in formulas according to indications. However, Ginseng Decoction (which also contains licorice) is known to cause edema or rashes occasionally. Other formulas containing ginseng are virtually safe in this regard.

Ginseng should not be taken by persons with very high blood pressure (systolic reading > 180 mm Hg). It is unsuitable in general for sthenic patients and those presenting with significant signs of heat.

Licorice

Licorice is an ingredient in 70% of common Kampo remedies. It contains glycyrrhizin, which has been made into an anti-ulcer drug (carbenoxolone). This constituent and its aglycone, glycyrrhetinic acid, have an aldosterone-like activity and have induced pseudo-aldosteronism in some patients, with effects such as hypertension, hypokalemia, and edema.

Unconcentrated extract of the whole root has very low toxicity, but prolonged administration of large quantities may still cause edema and elevated blood pressure. The amount of licorice in most Kampo formulas does not exceed 3.0g. and is usually safe. The risk of adverse effects is greater with prolonged administration of a formula containing large amount of licorice (such as Peony and Licorice Decoction) or multiple formulas containing licorice; or with the concomittant use of diuretic drugs that cause excessive loss of potassium. The risk is reduced if the formula also contains Kampo diuretics such as atractylodes, poria, fangji, polyporus, and alisma.

---

[2]: *Many of these substances are diaphoretics rich in essential oils, known as exterior-resolvents (substances that resolve exterior patterns) in traditional medicine.*

Poria Five Powder may be prescribed to treat edema resulting from licorice overdose, but the condition will disappear on its own within a few days upon discontinuation of the medication.

Formulas containing more than 2.5g. of licorice are contraindicated in patients with aldosteronism, myopathy, or hypokalemia.

III. Nervous system effects

Aconite

Aconite is a poisonous root with analgesic, cardiotonic, and metabolic stimulating actions. The aconite used in Kampo extract preparations has been processed to greatly reduce its toxicity, and is relatively safe as long as it is used according to indication. However, overdose can still cause symptoms such as flushing, palpitations, sweating, light-headedness, numbness, and nausea.

Aconite is generally unsuitable for children and sthenic individuals, who are more susceptible to its adverse effects. It is contraindicated in patterns with significant heat signs. Avoid in pregnancy and in cases with heart block, myocardial disorders, or abnormal liver function.

Persons experiencing the mild toxic effects of aconite should immediately drink as much fluid as possible. A decoction of mung beans or mung beans with licorice is an effective traditional antidote for mild aconite poisoning. Atrophine injection is necessary for acute cases.

Remedies containing aconite are given for cold patterns and are typically taken warm. However, in cases of cold lower body accompanied by local heat signs in the upper body (such as flushing), it is better taken cold to avoid triggering adverse effects.

Ephedra

Ephedra contains the chemical ephedrine, which has a stimulating effect on the sympathetic nervous system and can cause excessive sweating, palpitations, cardiac arrhythmia, restlessness, and insomnia. Used judiciously, ephedra formulas rarely induce these symptoms. The risk increases if they are used with anti-cough medications containing ephedrine.

Ephedra may cause GI disturbances such as anorexia, epigastric pain, and diarrhea. It may also cause rashes or itching or worsen existing skin conditions in susceptible patients.

Administration is not suitable in hyperthyroidism, heart diseases, hypertension, kidney disorders, and prostate hypertrophy. Use with particular caution in the elderly, persons with digestive problems, and the asthenic in general. Avoid concomitant use of drugs with sympathomimetic actions.

IV. GI disturbances

This is the most common type of adverse effect associated with Kampo remedies. The following substances may cause gastric distress, anorexia, nausea, abdominal pain, or diarrhea:

Coptis

Gardenia

Gypsum – Extracts are less likely to cause problems than decoctions.

Ligusticum

Mirabilite – Avoid in persons prone to digestive disturbances, the elderly, and the asthenic in general.

Peach kernel

Rehmannia – Can cause GI disturbances on account of its cloying nature. Intermittent administration may be desirable if rehmannia is to be taken over long-term, as persons who tolerate it well initially can develop such symptoms after continuous chronic use. Perfect Major Supplementation Decoction and Honey-Fried Licorice Decoction contain rhemannia but rarely induce GI symptoms.

Rhubarb – Unsuitable in persons prone to digestive disturbances and the asthenic in general, in whom even a small quantity (<0.5g.) can precipitate such symptoms.

Spiny jujube

Tangkuei

Peony (in extract form or in decoction) may possibly cause constipation on account of its astringency.

Cinnamon and **Dried Ginger**[3] can possibly aggravate peptic ulcers. Extract preparations are safer than decoctions in this regard.

V. Excessive menstrual bleeding and pregnancy

Excessive menstrual bleeding

The following substances should be avoided:

Achyranthes

Carthamus

Ligusticum

Mirabilite – Avoid in general during menstruation

Moutan

Mutong

Peach kernel

Rhubarb – Avoid in general during menstruation

Cinnamon – Use with caution

Pregnancy

The following substances are traditionally contraindicated during pregnancy:

Achyranthes

Carthamus

Corydalis

---

[3] *In Japanese practice, many remedies formulated with fresh ginger may actually be prepared with dried ginger in lesser amounts.*

Moutan
Mutong
Peach kernel
Sappan
Unripe bitter orange

The following substances are to be avoided or used with caution:

Aconite
Cinnamon
Dried ginger[3]
Magnolia bark
Mirabilite – Avoid during pregnancy and the postpartum period
Pinellia
Rhubarb – Avoid during pregnancy and the postpartum period. Contraindicated in nursing mothers since active ingredients enter the milk.

The following substances stimulate the uterus experimentally and are best avoided during pregnancy:

Coix
Evodia
Magnolia flower
Spiny jujube kernel

In general, avoid all formulas with significant diaphoretic, diuretic, or laxative actions.

References for Appendix A

Nihon Seiyaku Dantai Rengōka (Alliance of Japanese Pharmaceutical Corporations), ed. *Ippanyō Kampō Seizai Shiyō jō no Chūi (Cautionary Notes on the Application of General-Use Kampo Preparations)*. Yakugyōjihōsha, 1989.

Kobe Chinese Medicine Research Society, ed. *Jōyō Kanyaku Handobuku (Handbook of Common Chinese Medicinal Substances)*. Tokyo: Ishiyaku Publishing Company, 1987.

Kobe Chinese Medicine Research Society. *Kanyaku no Rinshō Ōyō (Clinical Applications of Chinese Medicinal Substances)*. Tokyo: Ishiyaku Publishing Company, 1979.

Kikutani, Toyohiko. "Kampōyaku no Fukusayō (Side Effects of Kampo Medicine I & II)" . In *Nihon Yakuzaishikai Zasshi* (Journal of Japanese Pharmaceutical Association) 34:7,8, 1982.

Kikutani, Toyohiko et al. "Kampōyaku to Fukusayō (Kampo Medicine and Side Effects)". In *Kampō Hoken Shinryō Shishen*. Japan Society of Oriental Medicine, 1986, pp.32-34.

Bensky, Dan and A. Gamble. *Chinese Herbal Medicine, Materia Medica*. Seattle: Eastland Press, 1986.

---

[3] *See footnote 2.*

Appendix B

American Distributors of Kampo Prepared Medicines

Brion Herbs Corporation
12020-B Centralia Road
Hawaiian Gardens, CA 90716

Meridian Traditional Herbal
26 McGirr St.
Cumberland, RI 02864

Qualiherb
13340 E. Firestone Blvd., Suite N
Santa Fe Springs, CA 90670

Tashi Enterprises (Ming Tong)
3252 Ramona Street
Pinole, CA 94564

Selected Glossary of Technical Terms

Technical terms are rendered in accordance with *A Practical Dictionary of Chinese Medicine* when their significance in Kampo conforms closely to that in Chinese medicine. The glossary herein provides the translation and a brief definition of classical and modern terms that are either unique to Kampo or differ significantly in interpretation from their Chinese counterparts. Consult the text for more detailed discussions.

abdominal examination *(fukushin)* 腹診

Kampo-style diagnostic palpation of the abdominal wall. Findings of abdominal examination contribute to the determination of constitutional state and the identification of pathology in traditional terms, and suggest the pertinence of certain substances or formulas. Emphasized over pulse diagnosis in Kampo for chronic disorders.

abdominal sign *(fukukō, fukushō)* 腹候、腹証

A significant feature of the abdominal wall identified and interpreted in Kampo abdominal examination.

abdominal strength *(fukuryoku)* 腹力

A qualitative index evaluated through palpation of the abdominal wall. Characteristics such as thickness, resilience, good muscular development, and a fair deposit of subcutaneous fat contribute to a diagnosis of strength. Conversely, characteristics such as thinness, softness, poor muscular development, scant fat deposit, or obese flabbiness denote the lack of strength. Abdominal strength reflects the general fitness and nutritional status of the body.

asthenia *(kyo, kyosei taishitsu)* 虚、虚性体質

A frail or adynamic state; susceptible to pathologies characterized by hypotonus, hyporeaction, and insufficiency. The opposite of sthenia.

blood stasis abdominal signs *(oketsu no fukushō)* 瘀血の腹証

One or more loci of resistance and tenderness in the lower abdomen identified by palpation, signifying the presence of blood stasis pathology.

coldness syndrome *(hieshō)* 冷え症

Local or systemic chronic sensations of coldness, most commonly affecting the extremities and the lower torso.

constitutional state *(taishitsu)* 体質

A qualitative index of vigor and resistance against illness evaluated from individual factors such as body type, muscular development, healing response, predispositions and susceptibilities. In this book, constitutional state is codified by a 5-level ordinal scale:

5 = sthenic   4 = somewhat sthenic   3 = intermediate
2 = somewhat asthenic   1 = asthenic

fluid imbalance *(suishō, suidoku)* 水証、水毒

Any pathologic distribution, discharge, or stagnation of bodily fluids other than blood. More narrowly, refers to abnormal fluid stagnation and its clinical manifestations.

formula pattern *(hōshō, yakushō)* 方証、薬証

A cluster of symptoms and signs indicating treatment by a particular formula. Also functions as a basic unit of diagnosis in Kampo, where (in the Classical tradition) pathologic conditions are differentiated and categorized according to the appropriate means of treatment.

headrush *(jōshō, nobose)* 上衝、のぼせ

An uncomfortable sensation of heat, congestion, or mounting pressure in the upper body, especially in the head, often with visible flushing in the face.

headrush syndrome *(noboseshō)* のぼせ証

Headrush together with such symptoms as flushing, headache, palpitations, etc., that tend to occur in association with it.

healing crisis *(mengen)* 瞑眩

Transient acute reactions that may occur upon initiation of therapy and heralds the start of recovery.

hypotonic lower abdomen 臍下不仁、少腹不仁
(seika fujin, shōfuku fujin)

Relative softness in the center of the lower abdomen compared to other parts of the abdominal wall. Sometimes accompanied by a diminished sensitivity in the area.

left lower quadrant hypersensitivity *(shōfuku kyūketsu)* 少腹急結

An acute painful reaction elicited by a superficial palpation maneuver in the left lower quadrant.

periumbilical pulsation *(seibu no dōki)* 臍部の動悸

Pulsation around the umbilicus detected by laying the palm or fingers lightly on the wall. It may sometimes be felt subjectively, and is occasionally a purely subjective sensation.

periumbilical region *(seibu)* 臍部

The area circumscribing the umbilicus about two finger breadths in radius.

rectus tension *(fukuchokkin no kinchō)* 腹直筋の緊張

Abnormal tension of the rectus muscles. May be general or localized to the upper or lower segments:

    general rectus tension *(fukushi kōkyū)* 腹皮拘急

    upper rectus tension *(shinka shiketsu)* 心下支結

    lower rectus tension *(shōfuku kōkyū)* 　少腹拘急

sthenia *(jitsu, jissei taishitsu)* 実、実性体質

Robust; susceptible to pathologies characterized by hypertonus, hyper-reaction, and repletion. The opposite of asthenia.

subcostal distress 胸脇苦満、肋骨弓下の抵抗・圧痛
(kyōkyōkuman, rokkotsukyūka no teikō attsū)

Resistance and tenderness beneath the costal margin elicited by palpation. Furthermore, the fingers of the examiner encounter resistance when an attempt is made to push them upward from under the edge of the costal margin into the thoracic cavity. This maneuver also induces discomfort or pain accompanied by a suffocating sensation in the chest. Associated with a subjective feeling of oppression or distressful fullness around the costal arch (the so-called "bitter fullness in the chest and lateral costal region").

subcostal region *(rokkotsukyū kabu)* 　肋骨弓下部

A region designated in Kampo abdominal examination. A zone beneath the costal margin comparable to the left and right hypochondriac regions and a part of the epigastric region.

substernal hard glomus *(shinka hikō)* 心下痞鞕

Resistance and tenderness elicited in the substernal region, accompanied by subjective discomfort.

substernal region *(shinkabu)* 心下部

A region designated in Kampo abdominal examination. Comparable to the epigastric region, but extends farther down to about an inch above the umbilicus.

substernal splashing sound 　心下部振水音、胃内停水の腹証
(shinkabu shinsuin, inai teisui no fukushō)

The sound of fluid moving about when the upper abdominal wall is percussed with the finger tips.

upper body heat and lower body cold *(jōnetsu gekan)* 上熱下寒

In Kampo, generally refers to headrushes accompanied by cold lower extremities.

weak digestive function *(ichō kyojaku)* 　胃腸虚弱

Chronic susceptibility to indigestion, diarrhea, or other gastrointestinal problems.

Bibliography

I. Works recommended in the text

Bensky, Dan and A. Gamble. *Chinese Herbal Medicine: Materia Medica.* Seattle: Eastland Press, 1986.

Lark, Susan M. *The Menopause Self Help Book.* Berkeley: Celestial Arts, 1992.

Wiseman, N and A. Ellis. *Fundamentals of Chinese Medicine.* Brookline, MA: Paradigm Publications, 1995.

II. Japanese and Chinese sources

Chao Yuan-Fang. *Origin and Outcome of Disease (Zhu Bing Yuan Hou Lun).* Sui, 610.

Zhang Jie-Bin (Jing Yue). *Jing Yue's Complete Compendium (Jing Yue Quan Shu).* Ming, 1624.

Zhang Zhong Jing. *Essential Prescriptions of the Golden Coffer (Jin Gui Yao Lue).* Later Han, c.220.

_____. *Treatise on Cold Damage (Shang Han Lun).* Later Han, c.220.

III. English Sources

Bensky, Dan and A. Gamble. *Chinese Herbal Medicine: Materia Medica.* Seattle, WA: Eastland Press, 1986.

Bensky, Dan and R. Barolet. *Chinese Herbal Medicine: Formulas and Strategies.* Seattle, WA: Eastland Pres, 1989.

Lock, Margaret M. *East Asian Medicine in Urban Japan.* Berkeley: University of California Press, 1980.

_____, "Rationalization of Japanese Herbal Medication: The Hegemony of Orchestrated Pluralism." *Human Organization* 49:1, 1990.

Otsuka, Yasuo. "Chinese Traditional Medicine in Japan." In *Asian Medical Systems,* edited by Charles Leslie. Berkeley: University of California Press, 1977.

Wiseman N. *A Practical Dictionary of Chinese Medicine.* Brookline, MA: Paradigm Publications, 1997.

_____, *English-Chinese–Chinese-English Dictionary of Chinese Medicine.* Hunan, China: Hunan Science Press, 1995.

Wiseman, N. and A. Ellis. *Fundamentals of Chinese Medicine (revised edition).* Brookline, MA: Paradigm Publications, 1995.

IV. Japanese and Chinese language sources

中国古医書　Pre-Modern Literature

傷寒論	漢・張仲景		
金匱要略	漢・張仲景		
萬病回春	明・龔廷賢		

現代日本漢方医書　Modern Kampo Literature

皇漢医学	湯本求真	燎原書店（1979　復刻版）	1928
漢方後世要方解説	矢数道明	医道の日本社	1959
傷寒論解説	大塚敬節	創元社	1966
漢方診療医典	大塚敬節、矢数道明、清水藤太郎	南山堂	1969
漢方医学の基礎と診療	西山英雄	創元社	1969
漢方医語辞典	西山英雄	創元社	1971
漢方古方要方解説	奥田謙蔵	医道の日本社	1973
漢方診療三十年	大塚敬節	創元社	1976
漢方処方応用の実際	山田光胤	南山堂	1977
漢方治療の方証吟味	細野史郎	創元社	1978
漢方入門講座	龍野一雄	雄渾社	1978
傷寒金匱要方解説	龍野一雄	雄渾社	1978
漢方概論	藤平健、小倉重成	創元社	1979
漢薬の臨床応用	中山医学院編、神戸中医学研究会編訳	医歯薬出版株式会社	1979
長倉漢方雑話	長倉音蔵	長倉製薬株式会社	1979
金匱要略講話	大塚敬節	創元社	1979
浅田流漢方診療の実際	高橋道史	医道の日本社	1980
臨床応用漢方処方解説	矢数道明	創元社	1981
漢方処方類方鑑別便覧	藤平健	株式会社リンネ	1982
漢方医学十講	細野史郎	創元社	1982
中医処方解説	神戸中医学研究会編	医歯薬出版株式会社	1982
漢方医学大辞典	漢方医学大辞典編集委員会編	雄渾社	1983
エキス剤による漢方診療ハンドブック	桑木崇秀	創元社	1983
東洋医学入門	大塚恭男	日本評論社	1983
特集：更年期障害		現代東洋医学第6巻第3号	1985
勿誤薬室方函口訣釈義	長谷川弥人	創元社	1985
臨床医の漢方診療指針	長谷川弥人、大塚恭男編集	メジカルビュー社	1985
図説漢方処方の構成と適用	森雄材	医歯薬出版株式会社	1985
漢方保険診療指針	漢方保険診療指針編集委員会編	日本東洋医学会	1986
中医臨床のための常用漢薬ハンドブック	神戸中医学研究会編著	医歯薬出版株式会社	1987
臨床医のための漢方（基礎編）	松田邦夫、稲木一元	株式会社カレントテラピー	1987
薬局製剤漢方 194方の使い方	埴岡博、滝野行亮	薬業時報社	1988
漢方治療症例選集	緒方玄芳	現代出版プランニング	1988
免疫と漢方	丁宗鉄	谷口書店	1988
万病回春解説	松田邦夫	創元社	1989
一般用漢方製剤使用上の注意解説	日本製薬団体連合会安全性懇談会編	薬業時報社	1989
漢方と鍼灸の腹証（古今腹証新覧）	小川新、池田太喜男、池田政一	漢方の友社	1989
黙堂柴田良治処方集	柴田良治著、北山進三編	黙堂会	1989
新版漢方医学		日本漢方医学研究所	1990
症例から学ぶ和漢診療学	寺澤捷年	医学書院	1990
漢方医者の眼	寺師睦宗	医道の日本社	1990
漢方腹証講座	藤平健	緑書房	1991
精神科漢方治療ケース集	松橋俊夫	金剛出版	1991
漢方Ｑ＆Ａ	矢数道明編	日本醫事新報社	1991
日本漢方の病態観（上）（下）	中村謙介	漢方の臨床第38巻第6号、第7号	1991
東洋医学入門	森下宗司	谷口書店	1992
漢方治療のＡＢＣ	松田邦夫、稲木一元、佐藤弘編	日本医師会雑誌 108(5) 臨時増刊号	1992
漢方製剤の活用便覧	谿忠人	医薬ジャーナル社	1992
日本の漢方治療の現状と今後（33）	伊藤清夫	漢方の臨床第40巻第5号	1993

Index

vaginal pH, elevated: 113, 121

vaginitis: 116-119, 121, 135,
159, 161, 172, 174, 184, 186,
192, 204, 207, 218, 222, 230,
231, 234-236, 241

vision, blurred: 46

W

wax gourd seed: 222

weak digestive function: 41,
48-49, 52, 83, 85, 89, 92, 136,
148, 160, 162, 188, 192-193,
199, 231, 224-225, 227, 242,
250

weeping skin conditions: 226

wēn jīng tāng: 159

wēn qīng yǐn: 241

wheat: 197

white peony: 158, 162, 164,
168, 194, 202, 206, 207, 219,
221, 229, 237

wǔ lín sǎn: 182

wǔ líng sǎn: 216

X

xīn gān huǒ wàng: 42